MILADY STANDARD ESTHETICS: FUNDAMENTALS

Student Workbook

To be used with

Milady Standard Esthetics:
Fundamentals

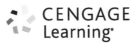

CENGAGE
Learning·

Australia • Brazil • Japan • Korea • Mexico • Singapore • Spain • United Kingdom • United States

CENGAGE
Learning·

Milady Standard Esthetics: Fundamentals Student Workbook, Eleventh Edition
Author: Jean Harrity

President, Milady: Dawn Gerrain

Director of Content and Business Development: Sandra Bruce

Acquisitions Editor: Martine Edwards

Associate Acquisitions Editor: Philip Mandl

Senior Product Manager: Jessica Mahoney

Editorial Assistant: Sarah Prediletto

Director of Marketing and Training: Gerard McAvey

Senior Production Director: Wendy A. Troeger

Production Manager: Sheron dra Thedford

Senior Content Project Manager: Nina Tucciarelli

Senior Art Director: Benjamin Gleeksman

For product information and technology assistance, contact us at
Cengage Learning Customer & Sales Support, 1-800-354-9706

For permission to use material from this text or product, submit all requests online at **www.cengage.com/permissions**
Further permissions questions can be emailed to
permissionrequest@cengage.com

Library of Congress Control Number: 2011943910

ISBN-13: 978-1-111-30691-5

ISBN-10: 1-111-30691-5

Milady
Executive Woods
5 Maxwell Drive
Clifton Park, NY 12065
USA

Cengage Learning is a leading provider of customized learning solutions with o ce locations around the globe, including Singapore, the United Kingdom, Australia, Mexico, Brazil, and Japan. Locate your local office at
www.cengage.com/global

Cengage Learning products are represented in Canada by Nelson Education, Ltd.

To learn more about Milady, visit **milady.cengage.com**

Purchase any of our products at your local college store or at our preferred online store **www.cengagebrain.com**

Printed at CLDPC, USA, 06-22

Contents

How to Use this Workbook / iv

1 History and Career Opportunities in Esthetics / 1

2 Life Skills / 12

3 Your Professional Image / 23

4 Communicating for Success / 28

5 Infection Control: Principles and Practices / 39

6 General Anatomy and Physiology / 54

7 Basics of Chemistry / 76

8 Basics of Electricity / 85

9 Basics of Nutrition / 94

10 Physiology and Histology of the Skin / 112

11 Disorders and Diseases of the Skin / 120

12 Skin Analysis / 133

13 Skin Care Products: Chemistry, Ingredients, and Selection / 145

14 The Treatment Room / 159

15 Facial Treatments / 167

16 Facial Massage / 180

17 Facial Machines / 187

18 Hair Removal / 195

19 Advanced Topics and Treatments / 207

20 The World of Makeup / 216

21 Career Planning / 232

22 The Skin Care Business / 242

23 Selling Products and Services / 256

How to Use this Workbook

This workbook has been especially designed to meet the needs, interests, and abilities of students receiving training for a career in esthetics, the art of skin care. It has been organized to be used in conjunction with *Milady Standard Esthetics: Fundamentals,* Eleventh Edition.

The material presented here has been prepared in accordance with the accepted methods of vocational training that are approved by state licensing organizations.

Mind mapping is used for developing an innovative and more creative approach to thinking. It simply creates a free-flowing outline of material or information. It is easy to learn, and when the technique is mastered, students will be able to organize an entire project or chapter in a matter of minutes. Mind mapping will allow students to release their creativity and engage both hemispheres of their brain. This technique has proved more effective than the linear form of note taking for most students. When mind mapping, the central or main idea is more clearly defined. The map lays out the relative importance of each idea or element of the subject matter. For example, the more important ideas or material will be nearer the center, and the less important material will be located in the outer parameters. Proximity and connections are used to establish the links between key concepts or ideas. The result is that review and recall will occur more quickly and be more effective. As you develop the art of mind mapping, you will see that each one takes on a unique appearance, which even adds to your recall ability of different topics or subjects. An example of how all the qualities, skills, and characteristics of an educator could be placed in a mind map is provided below.

1. Assignment and learning the Lesson

   The student writes the answers in the workbook, consulting the text and glossary located in the back of *Milady Standard Esthetics: Fundamentals,* Eleventh Edition.

2. Correction of the Lesson

   Answers may be corrected and/or rated during class or individual discussions or on an independent study basis.

3. Review of the Lesson

   Various tests emphasize the essential facts found in the textbook and measure the student's progress.

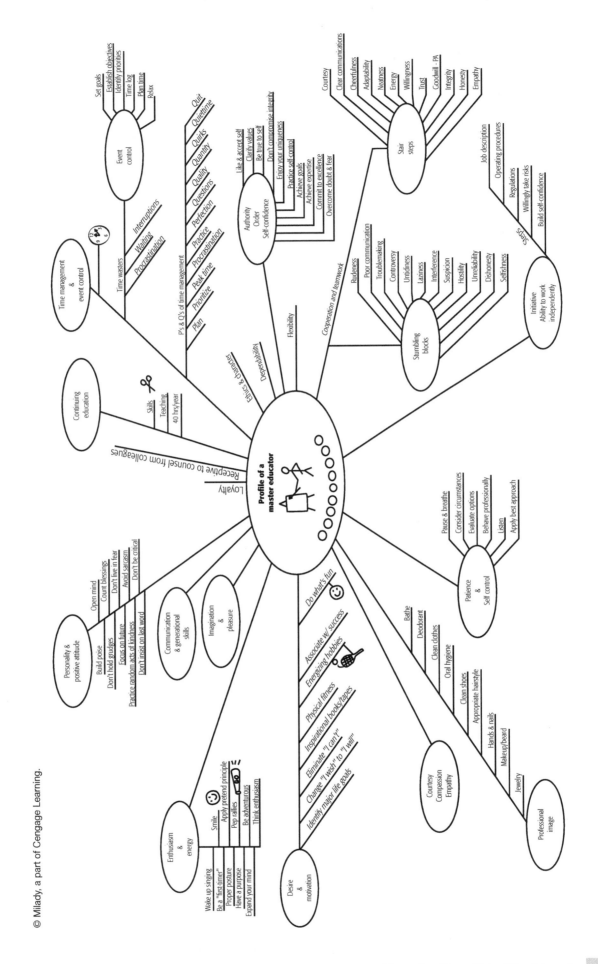

Profile of a master educator

Ethics & character

Dependability

Flexibility

Loyalty

Receptive to counsel from colleagues

Time management & event control

Event control
- Set goals
- Establish objectives
- Identify priorities
- Time log
- Plan time
- Relax

Time wasters
- Interruptions
- Waiting
- Procrastination

P's & Q's of time management
- Quit
- Quietime
- Quirks
- Quantity
- Quality
- Questions
- Perfection
- Practice
- Procrastination
- Peak time
- Prioritize
- Plan

Authority / Order / Self-confidence
- Like & accept self
- Clarify values
- Be true to self
- Don't compromise integrity
- Enjoy your uniqueness
- Practice self-control
- Achieve goals
- Achieve expertise
- Commit to excellence
- Overcome doubt & fear

Stair steps
- Courtesy
- Clear communications
- Cheerfulness
- Adaptability
- Neatness
- Energy
- Willingness
- Trust
- Goodwill - PA
- Integrity
- Honesty
- Empathy

Cooperation and teamwork

Stumbling blocks
- Rudeness
- Poor communication
- Troublemaking
- Controversy
- Untidiness
- Laziness
- Interference
- Suspicion
- Hostility
- Unreliability
- Dishonesty
- Selfishness

Initiative / Ability to work independently
- Job description
- Operating procedures
- Regulations
- Willingly take risks
- Build self-confidence

steps

Continuing education
- Skills
- Teaching
- 40 hrs/year

Personality & positive attitude
- Open mind
- Count blessings
- Don't live in fear
- Avoid sarcasm
- Don't be critical
- Build poise
- Don't hold grudges
- Focus on future
- Practice random acts of kindness
- Don't insist on last word

Communication & generational skills

Imagination & pleasure

Patience & Self control
- Pause & breathe
- Consider circumstances
- Evaluate options
- Behave professionally
- Listen
- Apply best approach

Do what's fun

Associate w/ success

Energizing hobbies

Physical fitness

Inspirational books/tapes

Eliminate "I can't"

Change "I wish" to "I will"

Identify major life goals

Professional image
- Bathe
- Deodorant
- Clean clothes
- Oral hygiene
- Clean shoes
- Appropriate hairstyle
- Hands & nails
- Makeup/beard
- Jewelry

Courtesy
Compassion
Empathy

Enthusiasm & energy
- Smile
- Apply pretend principle
- Pep rallies
- Be adventurous
- Think enthusiasm
- Wake up singing
- Be a "first-timer"
- Proper posture
- Have a purpose
- Expand your mind

Desire & motivation

CHAPTER 1 History and Career Opportunities in Esthetics

Date: _____

Rating: _____

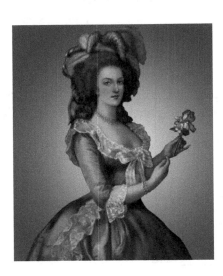

WHY STUDY HISTORY AND CAREER OPPORTUNITIES IN ESTHETICS?

Short Essay

Using the lines below, write down a description as to why you think it is important for you to learn about old and ancient techniques that were once used in skin care.

_____

_____

_____

_____

_____

_____

BRIEF HISTORY OF SKIN CARE

Fill in the Blank

Use the word bank below to fill in each blank with the appropriate word.

olive	scenery	rich oils
toothpicks	environment	baths
fingernails	kosmetikos	threading
temple	mignonette	tattooing
cosmetics	skin care	blackened

1. The Egyptians used _____ as part of their personal beautification habits, for religious ceremonies, and in preparing the deceased for burial.

2. Henna is obtained from the powdered leaves and shoots of the _____ tree.

3. Henna was used to dye hair and _____.

4. The early Hebrews had a wealth of grooming and _____ techniques.

5. The Hebrews used _____ and grapeseed oils to moisten and protect the skin.

6. The word *cosmetics* and *cosmetology* come from the Greek word

   _____.

7. The Greeks viewed the body as a _____.

8. The ancient Romans are famous for their _____.

9. After bathing, Romans applied _____ and other preparations to their skin to keep it healthy and attractive.

10. Both the Chinese and Japanese cultures blended the edges of their natural _____ into their looks.

11. Geishas removed their body hair by a technique similar to what we call _____ today.

12. From the tenth to the nineteenth centuries in the Asian culture, _____ teeth were considered beautiful and appealing.

13. Africans have created remedies and grooming aids from the materials found in their natural _____.

14. In North Africa, people use twigs from the mignonette tree as _____.

STYLE, SKIN CARE, AND GROOMING THROUGHOUT THE AGES

Matching

Match the time period clue on the left to the time period on the right.

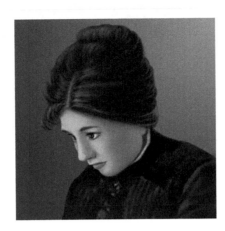

1. The period in European history between classical antiquity and the Renaissance.

_____

2. Marie Antoinette was queen of France from 1755 to 1793.

_____

3. It has brought about many changes in style, skin care, and innovations of the beauty culture.

_____

4. Spans the reign of Queen Victoria of England (1837–1901).

_____

5. This has a more relaxed approach to clothing, hair, and makeup.

_____

The Twenty-First Century

Middle Ages

The Age of Extravagance

The Twentieth Century

The Victorian Age

PRIVATE LABELING AND BRANDING

Create your own private label for your line of products using the space below. What would you call it? Which products would you have in your line? What would your logo look like?

```




```

_____

_____

_____

_____

_____

CAREER PATHS FOR AN ESTHETICIAN
Short Essay

In your own words, explain the job tasks for each position. Discuss your answers with your instructor. The first line is filled in for you to help get you started.

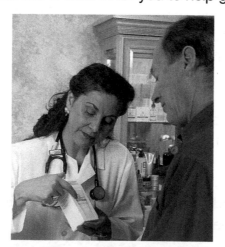

1. Salon or day spa esthetician

- Retailing

_____

_____

_____

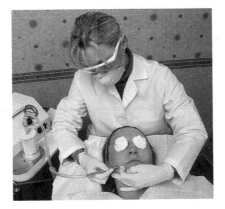

2. Medical aesthetician
- Microdermabrasion

_____

_____

_____

_____

_____

3. Destination spa
- Retailing

_____

_____

_____

_____

_____

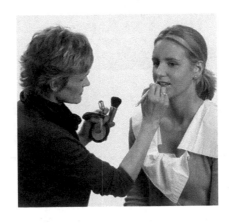

4. Makeup artist

• Applying concealer and foundation

_____

_____

_____

_____

5. Manufacturer's representative

• Learning the product ingredients

_____

_____

_____

_____

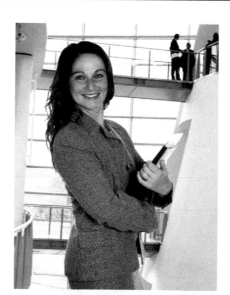

6. Cosmetics buyer

• Making cold calls

_____

_____

_____

_____

7. Beauty writer or editor
  • Reading text

_____

_____

_____

_____

_____

8. Esthetician on a cruise ship
  • Retailing

_____

_____

_____

_____

_____

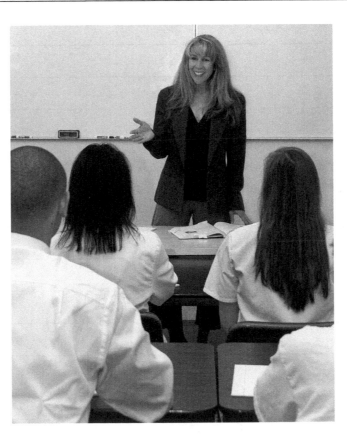

9. Educator

- Writing a curriculum

_____

_____

_____

_____

_____

A BRIGHT FUTURE

Short Essay

Estheticians taking a role in their local government also have an important job. One can become a state licensing inspector or examiner or a state board member. Create a list of what inspectors might look for upon entering a salon. You may need to research your own state's laws and regulations to obtain more information.

- Cleanliness

_____

_____

_____

_____

_____

1. A state board member also assists in creating and enforcing laws. Explain other tasks that he or she accomplishes.

_____

_____

_____

_____

_____

2. Now that your education has begun, explain where you would like to see your career in esthetics go. Would you want to be a medical aesthetician, day spa esthetician, or some other type? Explain why you are choosing that path.
Note: At the end of your education, look back to see what you wrote—do you feel the same, or did your ambition change?

_____

_____

_____

_____

_____

CAREER PATHS FOR AN ESTHETICIAN

Fill in the Blank

Fill in the blanks below with the appropriate answers.

1. Esthetics comes from the Greek word _____, meaning perceptible to the senses.

2. Estheticians offer skin care treatments and sell cosmetics but cannot prescribe _____ or give medical _____.

3. An esthetician is a person devoted to, or professionally occupied with, the _____ and _____ of the skin.

4. Estheticians in a salon or day spa are skin care _____ and _____.

5. Medical aesthetics involves the integration of _____ and _____.

6. A good makeup artist is skillful at _____ a person's more attractive features and _____ less attractive features.

7. Cosmetic manufacturers often hire _____ to call on salons or stores to sell products and help build clienteles.

8. Cosmetics _____ estimate the amount of stock an operation will need over a particular period and keep records of product purchases and sales.

9. Educators may teach esthetics in _____, _____, _____, or _____ schools.

10. Skin care products are continuing to become more _____ and have more efficient _____ that penetrate deeper into the skin.

11. Skin care in general is becoming more _____ than corrective.

12. The branch of anatomical science dealing with the health and well-being of the skin is called _____.

13. The field that integrates surgical and esthetic treatments is called

_____.

14. The medical setting in which patients receive both spa services and medical procedures is called a _____.

15. When you apply makeup to cover scars or congenital defects, you are performing _____.

16. A makeup artist who works in a mortuary is skilled at _____.

17. The travel industry is now using _____ for airport and in-flight services as well as on cruise ships.

18. Manufacturers often employ estheticians as _____ who conduct seminars and workshops, display products at conventions, and talk with teachers about the merits of the products.

19. Licensing exams are conducted and licenses are granted by

_____.

20. Americans born between the years 1946 and 1964 are known as

_____.

21. The U.S. Department of Labor predicts the rapid growth of _____ and a growing demand for practitioners licensed to provide a _____.

CAREER PATHS FOR AN ESTHETICIAN RAPID REVIEW TEST

Matching

Match the following terms with the most accurate description.

Term	Answer	Description
a) Estheticians in a spa or salon	_____	1. Demonstrate products to potential customers
b) Medical aestheticians	_____	2. Demonstrate products, cashiering
c) Salespeople/sales managers	_____	3. Serve the traveling public
d) Makeup artists	_____	4. Work for a magazine or newspaper

e) Manufacturer's reps	_____	5. Travel frequently; estimate stock for customers
f) Researchers	_____	6. Perform waxing and facial services
g) Cosmetics buyers	_____	7. Work in public, industrial, and vocational schools
h) Esthetics writers/editors	_____	8. Conduct regular salon inspections
i) Travel industry	_____	9. Determine the safety of products
j) Educators	_____	10. Work for television and movie productions
k) State licensing examiners	_____	11. Provide camouflage makeup and advanced treatments
l) State board members	_____	12. Conduct licensure examinations

IMPORTANT TERMS

Word Scramble

Unscramble each word by using the definition as a clue.

ehtsetaicin

1. A specialist in the cleansing, beautification, and preservation of the health of skin on the entire body, including the face and neck. _____

ethsecits

2. A branch of anatomical science that deals with the overall health and well-being of the skin, the largest organ of the human body. _____

nnaeh

3. A dye obtained from the powdered leaves and shoots of the mignonette tree; used as a reddish hair dye and in tattooing. _____

ledimac ashetsceti

4. The integration of surgical procedures and esthetic treatments. _____

nonachtelonoyg

5. The art of manipulating materials on an atomic or molecular scale. _____

CHAPTER 2 Life Skills

Date: _____

Rating: _____

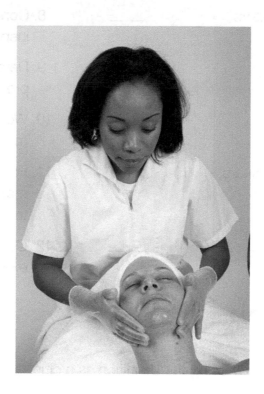

WHY STUDY LIFE SKILLS?

Short Essay

As an esthetician, your primary job responsibility is promoting skin health and beauty. To be successful in this people-oriented business, you will need excellent life skills. List some life skills that would like to learn and practice. Why are these life skills important to you? Use the lines below for your answer.

_____

_____

_____

_____

_____

THE PSYCHOLOGY OF SUCCESS

Short Essay

In your own words, explain what the following guidelines mean to you using the lines beneath each guideline.

1. Build Self-Esteem

_____

_____

_____

_____

_____

2. Visualize Your Success

_____

_____

_____

_____

_____

3. Build on Your Strengths

_____

_____

_____

_____

_____

4. Learn from Your Mistakes

_____

_____

_____

_____

_____

5. Define Success for Yourself

_____

_____

_____

_____

6. Practice Your Presentation Skills

_____

_____

_____

_____

_____

7. Develop Good Networking Skills

_____

_____

_____

_____

_____

8. Keep Your Personal Life Separate from Your Work

_____

_____

_____

_____

_____

9. Keep Your Energy Up (How can you do that?)

_____

_____

_____

_____

_____

10. Respect Others

_____

_____

_____

_____

_____

11. Stay Productive (How do you stay productive? When you don't feel like you are being productive, what are some motivational techniques that you use to help yourself?)

_____

_____

_____

_____

_____

STUDY SKILLS

Short Essay

Answer the questions on the lines provided.

1. Explain what your study skills are now. Do you study in your room? In the dining room? At a coffee shop?

_____

_____

_____

_____

_____

2. Is what you are doing now working?

_____

3. How can adapting some of these pointers assist you in your study habits? What will you change?

_____

_____

_____

_____

_____

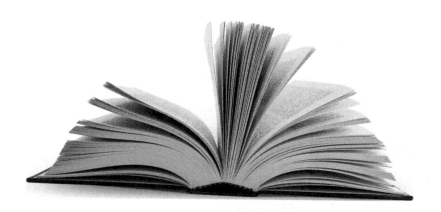

MISSION STATEMENT

Short Essay

Every company has a mission statement. They are words that everyone lives by. Every person that has a resume usually uses the objective as the mission statement. Create your mission statement and explain what it means to you using the lines below.

_____

_____

_____

_____

_____

GOAL SETTING

Short Answer

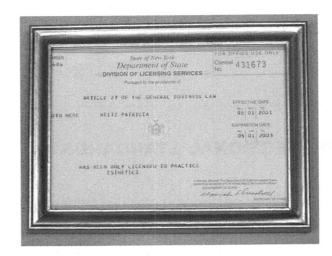

Complete the lists below with the tasks or events in your life that you would like to accomplish within the specified time frame.

1. Within the next 12 months? (Example: finish my esthetics course and apply for my state board)

_____

_____

_____

_____

_____

2. Within the next five years? (For example: Work in a successful salon and build a clientele, have children, etc.)

_____

_____

_____

_____

_____

3. Within the next 10 years? (For example: own my own salon and go skydiving).

_____

_____

_____

_____

_____

MANAGING PROFESSIONAL STANDARDS

Fill in the Blank

List the general guidelines that will help you maintain credibility and build confidence. A few guidelines are filled in for you.

1. Obtain the necessary credentials to practice in your state.

2. _____

_____

_____

_____

3. _____

_____

_____

_____

4. Show respect for your colleagues and supervisors. Do not make derogatory comments about other practitioners or undermine your employer's policies and price structure.

5. _____

_____

_____

_____

6. _____

_____

_____

_____

7. Be honest and truthful. Do not make false claims about products and techniques. When you do not have the answer, simply say, "I don't know, but I'll find out for you."

8. _____

_____

_____

_____

_____

9. Be open to seeking consultation from more experienced colleagues or other professionals.

10. _____

_____

_____

_____

_____

ATTITUDE

True/False

Identify the following statements as either true or false.

True/False   **1.** Being critical and vague in dealing with others is an example of diplomacy.

_____

True/False   **2.** Displaying self-control and maturity is an example of emotional stability.

_____

True/False   **3.** Being interested in other people's feelings, opinions, and ideas is an example of receptivity.

_____

True/False   **4.** Lack of concern and responsiveness and acting overly critical are examples of sensitivity.

_____

True/False   **5.** Your behavior, including your manners and your judgment, is an example of values and goals.

_____

True/False

6. Communication skills do not require an understanding of people's needs and desires.

_____

True/False

7. Not disclosing personal information of a client is the responsibility of the esthetician as well as an example of discretion and confidentiality.

_____

True/False

8. A way to maintain boundaries is to remember that an esthetician is also a counselor.

_____

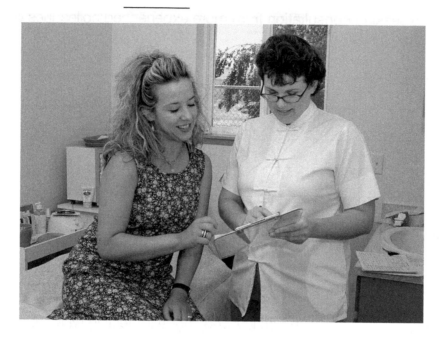

MOVING FORWARD IN YOUR CAREER

Word Search

Write the correct term next to its definition on the lines below. Once you have identified these terms, find them in the word search on page 21.

Word	Clue
_____	The moral principles by which we live and work.
_____	The conscious act of planning your life rather than just letting things happen.
_____	The identification of long- and short-term goals that helps you decide what you want out of life.
_____	A statement that establishes the values that an individual or institution lives by as well as future goals.

_____ An unhealthy compulsion to do things perfectly.

_____ To make a list of tasks that need to be done in the order of most to least important.

_____ Putting off until tomorrow what you can do today.

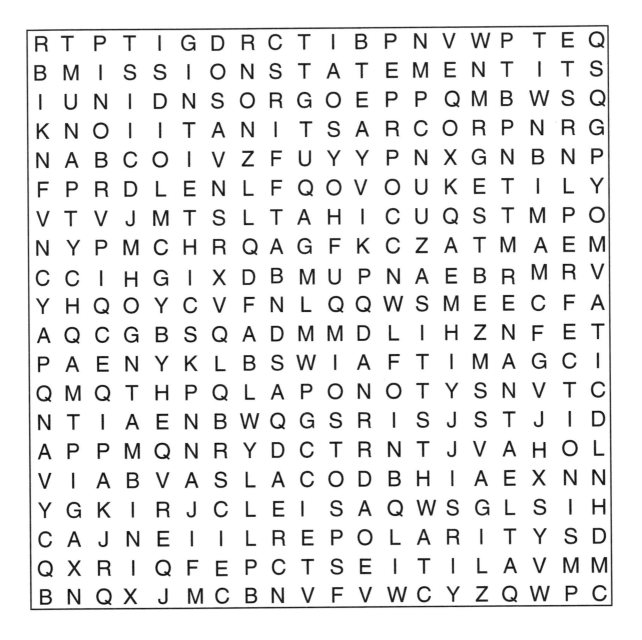

```
R T P T I G D R C T I B P N V W P T E Q
B M I S S I O N S T A T E M E N T I T S
I U N I D N S O R G O E P P Q M B W S Q
K N O I I T A N I T S A R C O R P N R G
N A B C O I V Z F U Y Y P N X G N B N P
F P R D L E N L F Q O V O U K E T I L Y
V T V J M T S L T A H I C U Q S T M P O
N Y P M C H R Q A G F K C Z A T M A E M
C C I H G I X D B M U P N A E B R M R V
Y H Q O Y C V F N L Q Q W S M E E C F A
A Q C G B S Q A D M M D L I H Z N F E T
P A E N Y K L B S W I A F T I M A G C I
Q M Q T H P Q L A P O N O T Y S N V T C
N T I A E N B W Q G S R I S J S T J I D
A P P M Q N R Y D C T R N T J V A H O L
V I A B V A S L A C O D B H I A E X N N
Y G K I R J C L E I S A Q W S G L S I H
C A J N E I I L R E P O L A R I T Y S D
Q X R I Q F E P C T S E I T I L A V M M
B N Q X J M C B N V F V W C Y Z Q W P C
```

© Milady, a part of Cengage Learning.

PROCRASTINATION

Short Essay

Draw on your past experiences to answer the questions below.

In the past, what did you procrastinate about? Did you ever accomplish that goal? If you did accomplish that goal, what was it? If you have not yet accomplished that goal, what is preventing you from doing so?

_____

_____

_____

_____

_____

CHAPTER 3 Your Professional Image

Date: _____

Rating: _____

WHY STUDY YOUR PROFESSIONAL IMAGE?

Short Essay

What are five important points when you are trying to portray a professional image?
Use the space provided to write down your points.

- _____
  _____

- _____
  _____

- _____
  _____

- _____
  _____

- _____
  _____

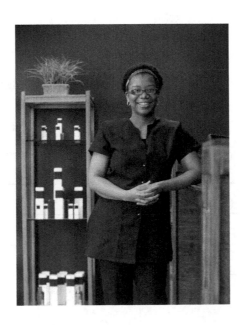

YOUR PROFESSIONAL IMAGE

Fill in the Blank

Fill in the blanks with an answer.

1. The impression projected by a person engaged in any profession.

   _____

2. Your professional image is made up of your _____ and your _____ in the workplace.

3. If you do not _____, your clients will assume that you cannot make them _____.

4. Personal hygiene is the daily maintenance of _____ and _____ through certain sanitary practices.

5. Personal hygiene consists of certain basic tasks, including:

   a) _____

   b) _____

   c) _____

   d) _____

   e) _____

   f) _____

   g) _____

6. Your posture, movements, and the way you walk make up your

   _____.

7. Good posture can prevent _____ and other physical problems.

8. To achieve good standing posture, practice these six steps:

   a) _____

   b) _____

   c) _____

   d) _____

   e) _____

   f) _____

9. To achieve good sitting posture, take these four steps:

a) _____

b) _____

c) _____

d) _____

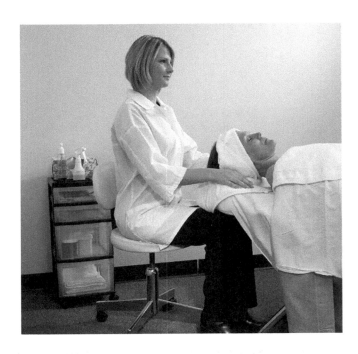

ERGONOMICS

Short Answer

Answer the following questions on the lines that are provided for you.

1. Define the term *ergonomics*.

_____

_____

_____

_____

_____

2. Using the blank space below, name or draw some of the items that can be ergonomically correct in your workspace. You can also utilize magazines and photos to cut and paste into the space.

PROFESSIONAL CONDUCT: SELF REFLECTION

Short Essay

There are a few questions to ask yourself to be sure that you are conducting yourself professionally. After reading the question, recite a time where the answer to the question was negative. On the lines below, explain how you reacted at that time and then explain what you could have done differently.

1. Am I warm, pleasant, and friendly to each person that I come in contact with?

_____

_____

_____

_____

_____

2. Do I maintain appropriate boundaries and treat even the most benign client information as privileged?

_____

_____

_____

_____

_____

3. Do I keep my ego in check and compromise as needed to maintain professional relationships?

_____

_____

_____

_____

_____

MASTERING SELF CONTROL

Fill in the Blank

Answer the following question on the lines below.

What are the eight suggestions to follow when a conflict arises?

1. _____

2. _____

3. _____

4. _____

5. _____

6. _____

7. _____

8. _____

CHAPTER 4 Communicating for Success

Date: _____

Rating: _____

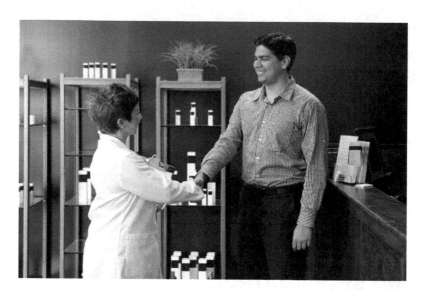

© Milady, a part of Cengage Learning. Photography by Dino Petrocelli.

WHY STUDY COMMUNICATING FOR SUCCESS?

Short Essay

Estheticians work face to face with clients—a distinct advantage in determining their needs, wants, likes, and dislikes. To make the most of this prime time together, estheticians must have excellent communication skills. Communicating effectively is the basis of all long-lasting relationships with clients and co-workers. Explain how communicating effectively would benefit you on the lines below.

_____

_____

_____

_____

_____

COMMUNICATING FOR SUCCESS

Short Essay

Define of each of the following terms in your own words.

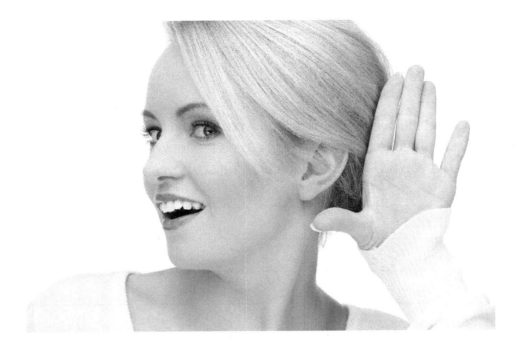

1. Client consultation:

   _____

   _____

   _____

2. Communication:

   _____

   _____

   _____

3. Consent form:

   _____

   _____

   _____

4. Reflective listening:

_____

_____

_____

CRITICAL THINKING

Short Essay

Explain in the lines below the last time you were in a difficult situation or were interacting with someone who was difficult to deal with. What did you do? How did you react? Could you have reacted differently? If so, how?

_____

_____

_____

_____

_____

HUMAN RELATIONS

Short Answer

List the 18 golden rules of human relations.

1. _____

_____

2. _____

_____

3. _____

_____

4. _____

_____

5. _____

_____

6. _____

_____

7. _____

_____

8. _____

_____

9. _____

_____

10. _____

_____

11. _____

_____

12. _____

_____

13. _____

_____

14. _____

_____

15. _____

_____

16. _____

_____

17. _____

_____

18. _____

_____

POSITIVE AND NEGATIVE NONVERBAL CUES

Fill in the Blank

Place each non-verbal clue under the correct category in the table provided.

NONVERBAL CUES

A frown	Using hand gestures to scold or embarrass
A pleasant tone of voice	A smile
Rapid and jumbled speech	Good eye contact
Appropriate body distance	A moderate tone of voice
A soft and unassertive voice	A simple nod to demonstrate you are listening
The gentle touch of a hand	A loud voice
Yawning, fidgeting with pens and paperclips, or other distracting gestures	Standing uncomfortably close to a person
Pursing the lips or folding arms in an off-putting manner	Warm and enthusiastic facial gestures
Looking away from a person	An even rate of speech

Positive Cues	Negative Cues

THE 10-STEP CONSULTATION METHOD

Fill in the Blank

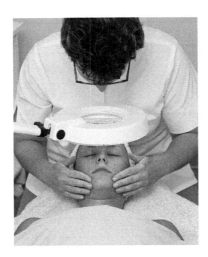

Below are the 10 rules to follow during a consultation. The terms are followed by the explanation. Fill in the missing part of each rule. The first rule has been completed for you.

1. REVIEW: Review the intake form that your client has filled out, and take a few minutes to develop rapport with the client and get the consultation going.

2. ASSESS: _____

   _____

   _____

   _____

   _____

3. _____ Ask your client what skin care products he or she is currently using. Does he or she love the fact that he or she only has to spend 10 minutes a day taking care of his or her skin? What professional treatments has he or she had in the past? Was he or she happy with the results? What is the reason for today's visit?

4. ANALYZE: _____

   _____

   _____

   _____

   _____

5. LIFESTYLE: _____

_____

_____

_____

_____

_____

_____

_____

_____

6. SHOW AND TELL: _____

_____

_____

_____

_____

_____

_____

_____

_____

_____

7. SUGGEST: Once you have enough information to make valid suggestions, narrow the treatment options based on the following four factors:

Lifestyle. _____

_____

_____

Skin type. _____

_____

_____

Skin conditions. _____

_____

_____

Fitzpatrick typing. _____

_____

_____

8. SUN EXPOSURE: Instructions regarding proper sun protection should be part of every consultation service. Use the Fitzpatrick scale to recommend the appropriate level of sun protection products and caution all clients against the harmful effects of overexposure to the sun. Estheticians should stress to clients that overexposure to the sun may not only lead to skin cancer but can also contribute to aging, hyperpigmentation, capillary damage, free-radical damage, and collagen and elastin deterioration. It is especially important to advise clients who have exfoliating treatments to keep out of the sun to avoid serious side effects.

9. MAINTENANCE: _____

_____

_____

_____

_____

_____

_____

10. REPEAT: _____

_____

_____

_____

_____

_____

_____

IN-SALON COMMUNICATION

Short Essay

Write your answer below using the lines that are provided for you.

In your own words, write down the eight guidelines to keep in mind while interacting and communicating with the staff.

1. _____
   _____
   _____
   _____
   _____
   _____
   _____
   _____

2. _____
   _____
   _____
   _____
   _____
   _____
   _____
   _____
   _____
   _____
   _____
   _____
   _____

3. _____
   _____
   _____
   _____

_____

_____

_____

_____

_____

_____

4. _____

_____

_____

_____

_____

_____

_____

_____

5. _____

_____

_____

_____

_____

_____

_____

6. _____

_____

_____

_____

_____

_____

_____

_____

_____

7. _____

_____

_____

_____

_____

_____

_____

_____

_____

_____

_____

8. _____

_____

_____

_____

_____

_____

_____

_____

_____

_____

_____

CHAPTER 5 Infection Control: Principles and Practices

Date: _____

Rating: _____

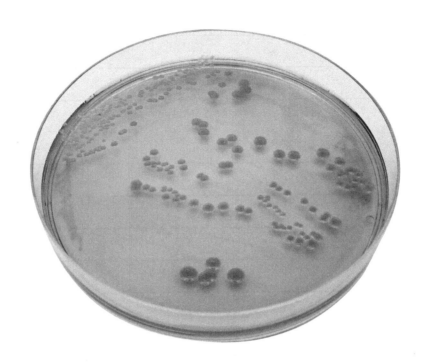

WHY STUDY INFECTION CONTROL: PRINCIPLES AND PRACTICES?

Short Essay

In your own words, describe why you feel estheticians should have a thorough understanding of infection control on the lines below.

_____

_____

_____

_____

_____

FEDERAL AGENCIES

Short Answer

Identify and describe each acronym.

1. OSHA:

_____

_____

_____

_____

_____

2. HCS:

_____

_____

_____

_____

_____

3. MSDS:

_____

_____

_____

_____

_____

PRINCIPLES OF INFECTION

Short Answer

Answer the following questions.

1. List the four organisms that are harmful to the body.

_____

_____

2. Define *pathogenic bacteria* below.

_____

_____

3. What are the routes of entry for pathogenic bacteria to enter the body?

- _____
  _____

- _____
  _____

- _____
  _____

- _____
  _____

- _____
  _____

4. In your own words, fill in the chart with the shape and the infection or disease it may cause.

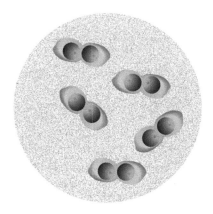

Bacteria	Shape	Infection/disease they may cause
Cocci	_____	_____
	_____	_____
	_____	_____
	_____	_____

Bacteria	Shape	Infection/disease they may cause
Staphylococci	_____	_____
	_____	_____
	_____	_____
	_____	_____
Streptococci	_____	_____
	_____	_____
	_____	_____
	_____	_____
Diplococci	_____	_____
	_____	_____
	_____	_____
	_____	_____
Bacilli	_____	_____
	_____	_____
	_____	_____
	_____	_____
Spirilla	_____	_____
	_____	_____
	_____	_____
	_____	_____

BASICS OF BACTERIA
Matching

Match the following words on the left with their definitions.

1. Bacilli

Organisms that grow, feed, and shelter on or in another organism (referred to as the host), while contributing nothing to the survival of that organism. _____

2. Bloodborne pathogens

Disease-causing microorganisms carried in the body by blood or body fluids. _____

3. Chelating soaps

Information compiled by the manufacturer about product safety, including the names of hazardous ingredients, safe handling and use procedures, precautions to reduce the risk of accidental harm or overexposure, and flammability warnings. _____

4. Contagious disease

An organism of microscopic or submicroscopic size. _____

5. Diagnosis

Detergents that break down stubborn films and remove the residue of products such as scrubs, salts, and masks. _____

6. Flagella

A ringworm fungus of the foot or athlete's foot. _____

7. HIV

The ability of the body to destroy and resist infection. Can be either natural or acquired and is a sign of good health. _____

8. Immunity

Human Immunodeficiency Virus _____

9. Infectious

Self-movement _____

10. MSDS

Determination of the nature of a disease from its symptoms and/or diagnostic tests. _____

11. Microorganism

Harmless microorganisms that may perform useful functions and are safe to come in contact with since they do not cause disease or harm. _____

12. Motility

Caused or capable of being transmitted by infection. _____

13. Non-pathogenic

Also known as communicable, a disease that is spread from one person to another person. _____

14. Non-porous

An item that is made or constructed of a material that has no pores or openings and cannot absorb liquids. _____

15. Parasites

Short, rod-shaped bacteria. They are the most common bacteria and produce diseases such as tetanus (lockjaw), typhoid fever, tuberculosis, and diphtheria. _____

16. Pathogenic

Abbreviated UP; a set of guidelines published by OSHA that require the employer and the employee to assume that all human blood and body fluids are infectious for bloodborne pathogens. _____

17. Personal protective equipment

The process that destroys all microbial life including spores. _____

18. Single use

Harmful microorganisms that can cause disease or infection in humans when they invade the body. _____

19. Spirilla

Also known as cilia; slender, hair-like extensions used by bacilli and spirilla for locomotion (moving about). _____

20. Sterilization

Abbreviated PPE; protective clothing and devices designed to protect an individual from contact with bloodborne pathogens; examples include gloves, fluid-resistant lab coat, apron, or gown, goggles or eye shield, and face masks that cover the nose and mouth. _____

21. Tinea pedis

Spiral- or corkscrew-shaped bacteria that cause diseases such as syphilis and Lyme disease. _____

22. Tuberculosis

A disease caused by bacteria that are transmitted through coughing or sneezing. _____

23. Universal Precautions

Also known as disposable; items that cannot be used more than once. These items cannot be properly cleaned so that all visible residue is removed or they are damaged or contaminated by cleaning and disinfecting in exposure incident. _____

DECONTAMINATION

Define the Term

Answer the following questions in the spaces provided.

1. Describe decontamination on the spaces below.

_____

_____

_____

2. Describe Decontamination Method #1 on the spaces below.

_____

_____

_____

3. Describe Decontamination Method #2 on the spaces below.

_____

_____

_____

4. Describe the difference between cleaning and sterilization on the spaces below.

_____

_____

_____

DISINFECTANTS

Short Answer

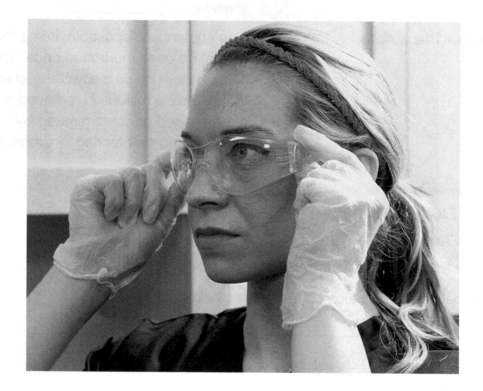

© Milady, a part of Cengage Learning. Photography by Paul Castle, Castle Photography.

List the 11 safety tips that you should remember when using disinfectants in the spaces provided.

1. Keep an MSDS on hand for the disinfectant(s) you use.

2. _____

_____

3. _____

_____

4. _____

_____

5. _____

_____

6. _____

_____

7. _____

_____

8. _____

_____

_____

9. _____

_____

_____

NEVER:

10. _____

_____

_____

11. _____

_____

_____

UNIVERSAL AND STANDARD PRECAUTIONS

Short Answer

Define and explain the following terms.

1. CDC:

_____

_____

_____

2. Universal Precautions:

_____

_____

_____

3. PPE:

_____

_____

_____

4. Standard Precautions:

_____

_____

_____

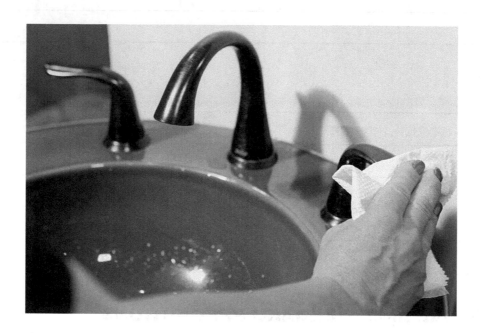

EXPOSURE INCIDENT

Fill in the Blank

What should you do if the client suffers from a cut or abrasion that bleeds during the service? List the 10 steps in the following spaces.

1. _____

_____

2. _____

_____

3. _____

_____

4. _____

_____

© Milady, a part of Cengage Learning. Photography by Dino Petrocelli.

5. _____

_____

_____

_____

6. _____

_____

_____

_____

7. _____

_____

_____

_____

8. _____

_____

_____

_____

9. _____

_____

_____

_____

10. _____

_____

_____

_____

PROFESSIONAL SALON IMAGE

Fill in the Blank

Fill in the missing guidelines for keeping your salon or spa looking its best.

- Keep floors and workstations dust free. Sweep hair off the floor after every client. Mop floors and vacuum carpets every day.

- _____
  _____

- Keep trash in a covered waste receptacle to reduce chemical odors and fires.

- _____
  _____

- Keep all work areas well lit.

- Clean and disinfect restroom surfaces, including door handles.

- _____
  _____

- Do not allow the salon or spa to be used for cooking or living purposes.

- Never place food in the same refrigerator used to store salon or spa products.

- _____
  _____

- Empty waste receptacles regularly throughout the day. A metal waste receptacle with a self-closing lid works best.

- _____
  _____

- _____
  _____

- Properly clean and disinfect all multiuse tools before reusing them.

- Store clean and disinfected tools in a clean, covered container. Clean drawers may be used for storage if only clean items are stored in the drawers. Always isolate used implements away from disinfected implements.

- _____
  _____

- _____
  _____

- Have clean, disposable paper towels for each client.

- Always properly wash your hands before and after each service.

- _____

_____

ACTIVITY

Use the blank space below to paste pictures of various items that would need to be cleaned and disinfected in a treatment room. You can find these pictures in magazines or on the Internet.

WORD REVIEW

Fill in the Blank

Insert the correct term in the space provided.

aseptic	dry heat	pathogens
asymptomatic	efficacy	sodium hypochlorite
contaminants	formalin	disinfected
decontamination	glass electrodes	antiseptic
double-bagging	immersion	Universal Precautions

1. Dirt, oils, makeup on a brush, or lotion on a cotton pad are all _____.

2. Removing pathogens from tools and surfaces is called _____.

3. Methods of sterilization include the autoclave and _____.

4. Tools that come into contact with blood or other bodily fluids must be _____.

5. Items such as _____ cannot be sterilized in an autoclave because they will break.

6. Any disinfectant used in a salon must have the correct _____ or effectiveness against pathogens.

7. _____ was used as a disinfectant in the past, but it is no longer considered safe for salon use.

8. The chemical term for household bleach is _____.

9. Proper disinfection procedure requires complete _____ in disinfectant for the required amount of time.

10. Handling sterilized and disinfected equipment and supplies so they are not contaminated until they are used on a client is called an _____ procedure.

11. In a blood spill, after cleaning the wound, apply an _____ to the wound.

12. Contaminated disposable objects such as cotton balls should be discarded by _____.

13. Sanitizing means significantly reducing the number of _____ on a surface.

14. OSHA prescribes the use of _____ as the approach to infection control.

15. A client who is _____ shows no symptoms or signs of infection.

KEY TERMS

Word Search

Using the word bank, find the words within the following word search.

aseptic	dry heat	pathogens
asymptomatic	efficacy	sodium hypochlorite
contaminants	formalin	disinfected
decontamination	glass electrode	antiseptic
double-bagging	immersion	Universal Precautions

```
U N I V E R S A L P R E C A U T I O N S
G A E K U A S Y M P T O M A T I C I S S
B Y R M E D O R T C E L E S S A L G O Q
J H T Q G C A C Y C A C I F F E N N D W
R A B G O V C Z F U Y Y P N X G O B I P
D D S D L T S L P Q O V R U K E I Q U Y
R O V T M Q S S T A H I D W S T S M M O
Y U D M N A R N S G T L M Z A P R A H M
H B I H G A X D I E U H N A M B E M Y V
E L S O Y M N F S L L Q O Q M E M C P A
A E I G B A Q I D M A E N G H T M F O T
T B N N Y K T B M W I M C T E M I G C I
Q A F T H Q A L A A D N R T Y N N V H C
N G E A G N B S Q V T R Q O R S S J L D
A G C B Q N R Y E C T N N T F O A H O L
V I T B I A S L A P V D O H I A D X R N
Y N E I R J C P E G T A Q C U G L E I H
C G D N Q I W T R E P I L A P F T Y T D
A N T I S E P T I C S E C T I Q A V E M
B W Q N O I T A N I M A T N O C E D P C
```

^{CHAPTER}6 General Anatomy and Physiology

Date: _____

Rating: _____

WHY STUDY GENERAL ANATOMY AND PHYSIOLOGY?

Short Essay

As an esthetic professional, an overview of human anatomy and physiology is part of your studies. What do you think the importance of anatomy and physiology is? Provide your answer on the lines below.

_____

_____

_____

_____

_____

THE CELL

Label the Image

Label the cell diagram with the following terms:

Nucleus, Cytoplasm, Cell membrane

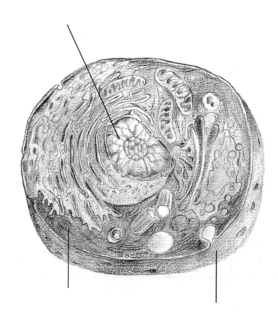

TISSUES

Short Answer

Cells make up tissues. List the four types of tissues below.

_____

_____

_____

_____

LIST SYSTEMS

Short Answer

Tissues make up organs and organs make up systems. The body systems engage certain organs that perform a specific function. There are 11 major systems in the body. List them below.

_____

_____

_____

_____

_____

_____

_____

_____

_____

_____

_____

THE SKELETAL SYSTEM

Fill in the Blank

Answer the following questions in the spaces provided.

1. How many bones are there in the skeletal system? _____

2. Bones are connected by movable and immovable _____.

3. Name the five primary functions of the skeletal system:

a) _____

b) _____

c) _____

_____

d) _____

e) _____

4. Elbows and knees are examples of _____ joints.

5. The skull is divided into two parts: the _____ and the _____ .

CRANIAL AND FACIAL BONES

Short Answer

There are 8 bones of the cranium and 14 facial bones. Define each of them in your own words.

Cranial Bones

1. Occipital bone (1):

_____

2. Parietal bones (2):

_____

3. Frontal bone (1):

_____

4. Temporal bones (2):

_____

5. Ethmoid bone (1):

_____

6. Sphenoid bone (1):

_____

Facial Bones

7. Nasal bones (2):

_____

8. Lacrimal bones (2):

_____

9. Zygomatic bones (2):

_____

10. Maxillary bones (2):

_____

11. Mandible bones (1):

_____

12. Turbinal bones (2):

_____

13. Vomer bone (1):

_____

14. Palatine bones (2):

_____

BONES OF THE NECK, SHOULDERS, AND BACK

Label the Image

Using the words from the following word bank, label the various parts of the diagram.

Clavicle	Hyoid	Sternum	Ribs
Cervical vertebrae	Scapula	Vertebrae	

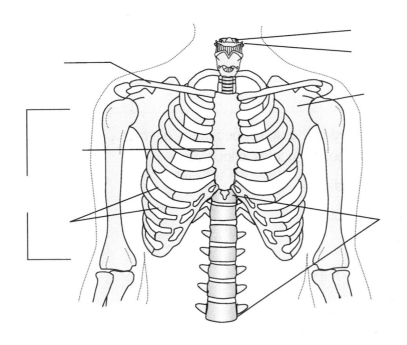
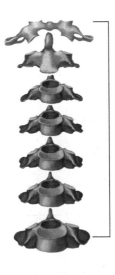

THE MUSCULAR SYSTEM

Short Answer

Answer the following questions in the spaces provided.

1. What are the main functions of the muscular system?

   a) _____

   b) _____

2. The body has more than 600 muscles, which account for approximately _____ percent of its weight.

3. What are the three types of muscle tissue?

   a) _____

   b) _____

   c) _____

4. The _____ is the part of the muscle that does not move.

5. The _____ is the part of the muscle at the more movable attachment to the skeleton.

6. Pressure in massage is usually directed from the _____ to the _____ .

7. List seven ways in which muscular tissue can be stimulated.

   a) _____

   b) _____

   c) _____

   d) _____

   e) _____

   f) _____

   g) _____

8. The following muscles are located in the scalp, neck, ear, eyebrow, nose, and mouth. Indicate where each of these muscles is located.

   a) _____: orbicularis oris

   b) _____: orbicularis oculi

   c) _____: frontalis

   d) _____: auricularis anterior

   e) _____: procerus

   f) _____: sternocleidomastoideus

Label the Image

9. Identify the muscles of the head, face, and neck in the corresponding spaces.
Once you have identified these muscles, label the image provided.

a) _____   i) _____

b) _____   j) _____

c) _____   k) _____

d) _____   l) _____

e) _____   m) _____

f) _____   n) _____

g) _____   o) _____

h) _____   p) _____

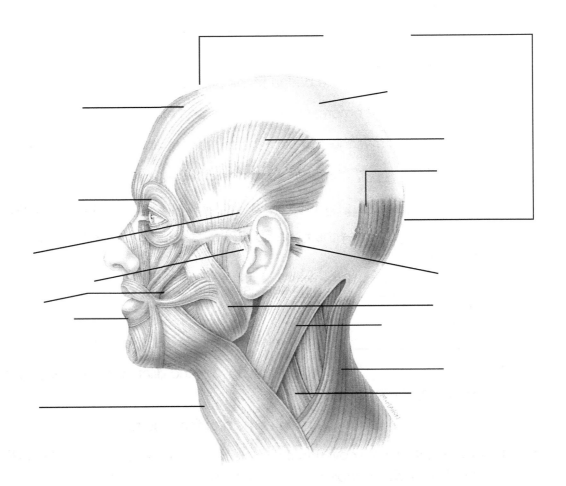

Fill in the Blank

Fill in the blanks using the word bank provided.

depressor labii inferioris	epicranius	serratus anterior
mentalis	levator labii superioris	procerus
chewing	corrugator	risorius
buccinators	auricularis	orbicularis oris
zygomaticus major/minor	triangularis	latissimus dorsi
levator anguli oris		

10. The _____ is the broad muscle that covers the top of the skull.

11. The _____ superior, anterior, and posterior are the muscles of the ear.

12. The masseter and temporalis muscles are sometimes referred to as the _____ muscles.

13. The eyebrow muscle that draws the eyebrow down and wrinkles the forehead vertically is the _____ muscle.

14. The _____ covers the bridge of the nose and lowers the eyebrows.

    a) _____ compresses the cheeks and expels air between the lips.

    b) _____ draws the corner of the mouth out and back, as in grinning.

    c) _____ compresses, contracts, puckers, and wrinkles the lips.

    d) _____ raises the angle of the mouth and draws it inward.

    e) _____ elevates the lower lip and raises and wrinkles the skin of the chin.

    f) _____ depresses the lower lip and draws it to one side.

    g) _____ elevates the lip, as in laughing.

    h) _____ elevates the lip and dilates the nostrils, as in expressing distaste.

    i) _____ pulls down the corners of the mouth.

16. The broad, flat muscle covering the back of the neck and upper and middle region of the back, controlling the shoulder blade, is called the _____.

17. The _____ is a muscle of the chest that assists in breathing and in raising the arm.

Matching

18. Match each of these muscles in the shoulder or arm to its description.

deltoid	supinator	triceps	extensors
biceps	flexors	pronators	

a) _____: wrist muscles involved in bending the wrist

b) _____: muscle producing the contour of the front and inner side of the upper arm

c) _____: muscles that straighten the wrist, hand, and fingers

d) _____: large muscle that covers the entire back of the upper arm and extends the forearm

e) _____: muscle that rotates the radius outward and the palm upward

f) _____: muscles that turn the hand inward so that the palm faces downward

g) _____: large, triangular muscle covering the shoulder joint

Label the Image

19. Identify the muscles of the shoulder and arm in the corresponding spaces. Once you have identified these muscles label the image provided.

a) _____   e) _____

b) _____   f) _____

c) _____   g) _____

d) _____

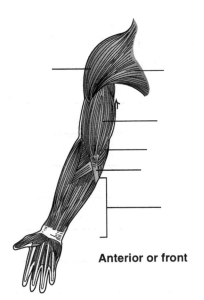

Anterior or front

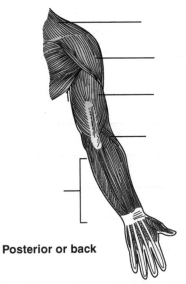

Posterior or back

© Milady, a part of Cengage Learning.

THE NERVOUS SYSTEM

Short Answer

Describe and define the different aspects of the nervous system.

1. The central nervous system: _____

_____

_____

_____

_____

2. The peripheral nervous system: _____

_____

_____

_____

_____

3. The autonomic nervous system: _____

_____

_____

_____

_____

BRAIN AND SPINAL CORD

Short Essay

The brain and the spinal cord are the main parts of the central nervous system.
There are four sections of the brain. Explain each of the sections in your own words.

1. Cerebrum: _____

_____

_____

_____

_____

_____

2. Cerebellum: _____

_____

_____

3. Diencephallon: _____

_____

_____

_____

_____

_____

_____

4. Brain stem: _____

_____

_____

_____

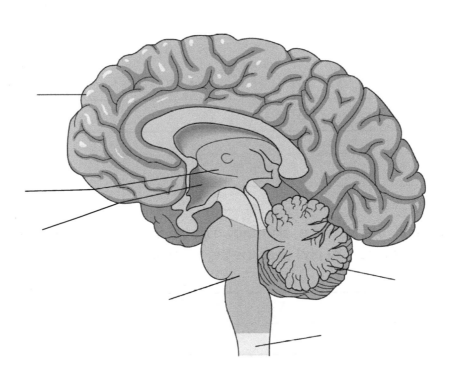

5. The fifth cranial nerve, also known as the trifacial or trigeminal, is the largest cranial nerve. List and briefly describe the various parts of this nerve.

- _____
  _____

- _____
  _____

- _____
  _____

- _____
  _____

- _____
  _____

- _____
  _____

- _____
  _____

- _____
  _____

- _____
  _____

- _____
  _____

6. The seventh cranial nerve, also known as the facial nerve, is the chief motor nerve of the face. List and describe the various parts to this nerve.

- _____

- _____

- _____

- _____

- _____

- _____

THE CIRCULATORY SYSTEM

Short Answer

Answer the following questions in the spaces provided.

1. What is the primary function of the circulatory system?

   _____

   _____

2. Name the two divisions of the circulatory system and their components:

   a) _____

   b) _____

   _____

3. What is the function of lymph? _____

   _____

4. What is the function of the heart? _____

   _____

Label the Image

5. Identify the parts of the heart in the corresponding spaces. Once you have
   identified the parts of the heart, label the image provided.

   a) _____

   b) _____

   c) _____

   d) _____

   e) _____

   f) _____

   g) _____

   h) _____

   i) _____

   j) _____

   k) _____

   l) _____

   m) _____

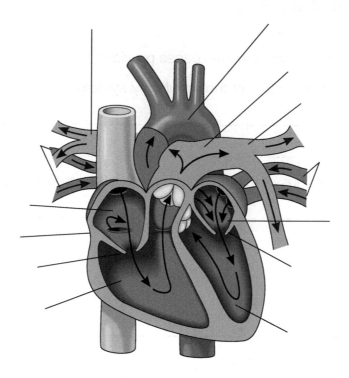

Short Answer

Answer the following questions in the spaces provided

6. The interior of the heart contains four chambers and _____ valves.

7. When the heart contracts and relaxes, blood flows in and then travels from the _____ to the _____ and out of the heart.

8. What is the normal heartbeat rate in a resting state? _____

9. Define the following terms.

   a) pulmonary circulation: _____

   _____

   b) systemic circulation: _____

   _____

   c) arteries: _____

   _____

   d) capillaries: _____

   _____

   _____

   e) veins: _____

   _____

   _____

Fill in the Blank

10. Fill in the blanks using the word bank provided.

corpuscles or cells	veins	hemoglobin
98.6°	8 to 10	83
arteries	platelets	plasma

    a) There are _____ pints in the human body.

    b) Blood is about _____ percent water.

    c) The normal temperature of blood is _____ Fahrenheit.

    d) Blood is bright red in the _____ and dark red in the _____.

    e) Blood is composed of red and white _____, _____, _____, and _____.

Short Answer

Answer the following questions in the spaces provided

11. Name the five primary functions of blood:

    a) _____

    _____

    b) _____

    _____

    c) _____

    _____

    d) _____

    _____

    e) _____

    _____

12. Red blood cells or corpuscles are produced in the _____.

13. Name the functions of these components of blood:

    a) red blood cells: _____

    b) white blood cells: _____

    c) platelets: _____

    d) plasma: _____

    _____

14. Lymph is filtered by lymph nodes, a process that helps fight _____.

15. Name the three primary functions of lymph:

a) _____

b) _____

c) _____

Label the Image

16. Identify the arteries of the head, face, and neck in the corresponding spaces. Once you have identified the arteries, label the image provided.

a) _____

b) _____

c) _____

d) _____

e) _____

f) _____

g) _____

h) _____

i) _____

j) _____

k) _____

l) _____

m) _____

n) _____

o) _____

p) _____

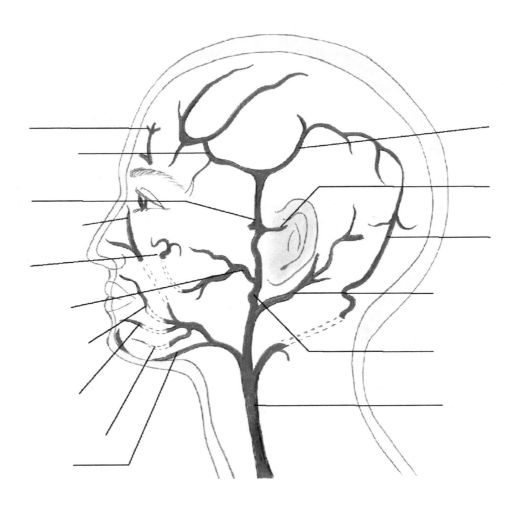

MATCHING

Match each of the following arteries with the area that it supplies blood to.

angular artery	transverse facial artery	posterior auricular artery
anterior auricular artery	middle temporal artery	infraorbital artery
superior labial artery	occipital artery	submental artery
parietal artery	frontal artery	
inferior labial artery	supraorbital artery	

a) _____: artery that supplies blood to the forehead and upper eyelids

b) _____: artery that supplies blood to the scalp, behind and above the ear

c) _____: artery that supplies blood to the upper eyelid and forehead

d) _____: artery that supplies blood to the upper lip and region of the nose

e) _____: artery that supplies blood to the side of the nose

f) _____: artery that originates from the internal maxillary artery and supplies blood to the eye muscles

g) _____: artery that supplies blood to the temples

h) _____: artery that supplies blood to the chin and lower lip

i) _____: artery that supplies blood to the skin and the masseter

j) _____: artery that supplies blood to the front part of the ear

k) _____: artery that supplies blood to the skin and muscles of the scalp and back of the head up to the crown

l) _____: artery that supplies blood to the side and crown of the head

m) _____: supplies blood to the lower lip

THE ENDOCRINE SYSTEM

Short Essay

There are two main glands within the body: exocrine and endocrine. Explain in your own words about the endocrine system including all of the glands within the system.

1. Endocrine system: _____

_____

_____

- _____

_____

_____

- _____

_____

_____

_____

- _____

_____

_____

_____

- _____

_____

_____

- _____
  _____
  _____

- _____
  _____
  _____

- _____
  _____

_____   _____

_____   _____

_____

_____

_____   _____

_____   _____

_____

_____

THE DIGESTIVE SYSTEM

Matching

Match the term with the correct definition.

_____ Peristalsis

_____ Digestion

_____ Absorption

_____ Defacation

1. elimination of feces from the body

2. moving food along the digestive tract

3. the transport of fully digested food into the circulatory system to feed the tissues and cells

4. breakdown of food by mechanical and chemical means

_____ Ingestion

5. responsible for breaking down foods into nutrients and wastes; consists of the mouth, stomach, intestines, salivary and gastric glands, and other organs

_____ Digestive enzymes

6. (eating or taking food into the body)

_____ Digestive system

7. (chemicals that change certain kinds of food into a form that can be used by the body)

THE EXCRETORY SYSTEM

Fill in the Blank

The body has various organs that remove waste products before they become toxic. Fill in the blank as to what the body rids itself of.

1. The kidneys excrete _____ .

2. The liver discharges _____ .

3. The skin eliminates _____ .

4. The large intestine eliminates _____ .

5. The lungs exhale _____ .

THE RESPIRATORY SYSTEM

Label the Image

Using the words from the word bank, label the following diagram.

| Nose | Left lung | Diaphragm | Right lung |

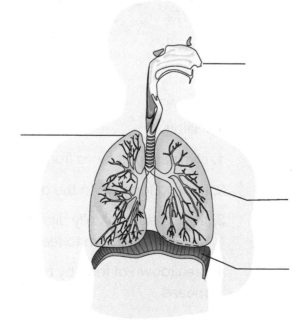

THE REPRODUCTIVE SYSTEM

Short Answer

Answer the following questions in the spaces provided.

1. What parts of the body are included in the reproductive system?

_____

_____

2. The reproductive system produces hormones—estrogen in females and testosterone in males. These hormones, or lack thereof, affect and change the skin in several ways as we age. List the ways hormones could affect the body.

_____

_____

ANATOMY AND PHYSIOLOGY KEY TERMS

Word Search

Place the corresponding word next to each of the definitions. Then identify the terms in the word search.

buccal nerve	femur	thorax	skin
dendrites	adipose tissue	ingestion	capillaries
hyoid bone	myology	epicranius	belly
abductors	axon	biceps	hemoglobin
melasma	lungs	occipitalis	lymph
diencephalon	clavicle	radius	absorption
supinator	tissue ulna	reflex	

1. Muscles that draw a body part, such as a finger, arm, or toe, away from the midline of the body or of an extremity. In the hand, these separate the fingers.

_____

2. The transport of fully digested food into the circulatory system to feed the tissues and cells. _____

3. A specialized connective tissue considered fat, which gives smoothness and contour to the body and cushions and insulates the body. _____

4. Sends impulses away from the cell body to other neurons, glands, or muscles.

_____

5. Middle part of a muscle. _____

6. Muscle producing the contour of the front and inner side of the upper arm. _____

7. Nerve that affects the muscles of the mouth. _____

8. Thin-walled blood vessels that connect the smaller arteries to the veins. _____

9. Also known as the collarbone; bone joining the sternum and scapula. _____

10. Tree-like branching of nerve fibers extending from a nerve cell; short nerve fibers that carry impulses toward the cell. _____

11. Located in the uppermost part of the midbrain; consists of two main parts, the thalamus and the hypothalamus. _____

12. Also known as the occipitofrontalis; broad muscle that covers the top of the skull. _____

13. Iron-containing protein in red blood cells that binds to oxygen. _____

14. U-shaped bone at the base of the tongue that supports the tongue and its muscle. _____

15. Eating or taking food into the body. _____

16. Spongy tissues composed of microscopic cells in which inhaled air is exchanged for carbon dioxide during one respiratory cycle. _____

17. Clear, yellowish fluid that circulates in the lymph spaces (lymphatic) of the body; carries waste and impurities away from the cells. _____

18. Condition of the skin that is triggered by hormones; causes darker pigmentation in areas such as on the upper lip and around the eyes and cheeks. _____

19. The study of muscles. _____

20. Back of the epicranius; muscle that draws the scalp backward. _____

21. Smaller bone in the forearm on the same side as the thumb. _____

22. Automatic nerve reaction to a stimulus; involves the movement of an impulse from a sensory receptor along the afferent nerve to the spinal cord, and a responsive impulse back along an efferent neuron to a muscle, causing a reaction. _____

23. External protective coating that covers the body. The body's largest organ; acts as a barrier to protect body systems from the outside elements. _____

24. Muscle of the forearm that rotates the radius out-ward and the palm upward. _____

25. Chest; elastic, bony cage that serves as a protective framework for the heart, lungs, and other internal organs. _____

26. Collection of similar cells that perform a particular function. _____

27. Inner and larger bone of the forearm, attached to the wrist on the side of the little finger. _____

```
D Q S A X O N E P E V R E N L A C C U B
R M B F E M U R A Q N O I T S E G N I S
A H E I D H Y U O I D B O N E E C C S U
D R L H S O R L Z J T V I E U P O L U P
I B L C O I Y Z Y U R Y U N C I N A Q I
U T Y D L M N G F B O S O A K C T V T N
S I C J P N O L U G S I P U Q R A I D A
P L R H C L W Q A I T I C N O A X C I T
N U M H O A X D T S L L I A C N E L E O
R N I Y Y T V E U L S B A T C I L E N R
S G M G S R S R A M O D A I I U F F C T
F S E K X O C R S L I M F T P S E G E S
B M I U P N I L G P S N H X I S R V P P
M N T I J E B O Q A S O A S T S T A H E
V H D T S N M Y L C R P N T A O Q H A C
P A F C V E B E A A C D B H L N W X L I
A E L I H J M L X B S A R E I A L S O B
A F A N L U E U S S I T L T S I B Y N A
M J R I Q F E D C N O I T P R O S B A V
L D E N D R I T E S F S R O T C U D B A
```

CHAPTER 7 Basics of Chemistry

Date: _____

Rating: _____

WHY STUDY CHEMISTRY?

Short Essay

Why should estheticians have a thorough understanding of chemistry? Provide your answer below.

_____

_____

_____

_____

_____

_____

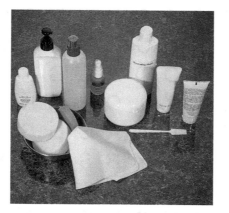

© Milady, a part of Cengage Learning. Photography by Larry Hamill.

CHEMISTRY

Short Answer

Answer the following questions in the spaces provided.

1. Why is it important for estheticians to have a basic knowledge of chemistry?

    a) _____

    _____

    b) _____

    _____

2. Define chemistry. _____

_____

_____

3. The two branches of chemistry are _____ and _____.

4. Organic chemistry studies substances that contain _____.

5. Gasoline, plastics, synthetic fabrics, pesticides, and fertilizers are manufactured from natural gas and oil and are therefore considered _____.

6. Metals, minerals, pure water, and clean air do not burn and are considered _____.

MATTER

Short Answer

Answer each question in the space provided.

1. Define matter. _____

2. What are the three forms of matter? _____

3. Give examples of physical properties. _____

_____

_____

4. What is an element? _____

_____

_____

5. What is an atom? _____

_____

_____

6. Describe a molecule. _____

_____

_____

7. Describe an elemental molecule. _____

_____

_____

8. Describe a compound molecule. _____

_____

_____

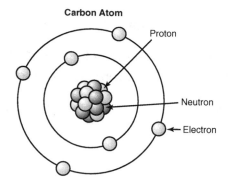

Carbon Atom

Proton

Neutron

← Electron

PHYSICAL AND CHEMICAL PROPERTIES OF MATTER

Short Answer

Define the following terms.

1. Physical properties: _____

_____

_____

2. Chemical properties: _____

_____

_____

3. Oxidation: _____

_____

_____

4. Physical change: _____

_____

_____

5. Chemical change: _____

_____

_____

MORE PROPERTIES OF MATTER

Fill in the Blanks

Fill in the blanks with the correct element from the clues provided.

water

1. It is a colorless, odorless, tasteless gas and is the _____ lightest element known. It is found in chemical combination with oxygen in water and with other elements in most organic substances.

nitrogen

2. It is the most abundant element found on Earth _____ and is a colorless, odorless, tasteless gas. It comprises about half of the Earth's crust, half of the rock, one-fifth of the air, and 90 percent of the water. It combines with most other elements to form an infinite variety of compounds, called oxides. One of the chief chemical characteristics of this element is its ability to support combustion.

hydrogen

3. It is a colorless, gaseous element. It makes up _____ about four-fifths of the air in our atmosphere and is found chiefly in the form of ammonia and nitrates.

oxygen

4. It is the gaseous mixture that makes up the _____ Earth's atmosphere. It is odorless and colorless and generally consists of about 1 part oxygen and 4 parts nitrogen by volume. It also contains a small amount of carbon dioxide, ammonia, and organic matter, which are all essential to plant and animal life.

air

5. It is the most abundant of all substances, _____ comprising about 75 percent of the Earth's surface and about 65 percent of the human body. Water is seldom pure. Natural spring water contains dissolved minerals, bacteria, and other substances.

POTENTIAL HYDROGEN (pH)

Label the Image

pH stands for potential hydrogen, which is a substance's relative degree of acidity or alkalinity and is measured on a scale of 0 to 14. The pH scale is a measure of the acidity and alkalinity of a substance; the pH scale has a range of 0 to 14, with 7 being neutral. A pH below 7 is an acidic solution; a pH above 7 is an alkaline solution.

1. Place the following items where they belong on the pH scale.

Lemon juice   Peroxide   Baking soda

Vinegar   Distilled water   Lye

Alum   Ammonia

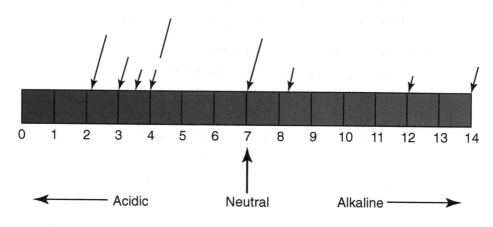

Short Answer

Define and describe the following terms.

2. Describe the oxidation-reduction reaction.

_____

_____

_____

_____

_____

_____

_____

_____

_____

_____

_____

_____

_____

3. Define combustion.

_____

_____

_____

4. Define antioxidants.

_____

_____

_____

_____

5. Define free radicals.

_____

_____

_____

CHEMISTRY AS APPLIED TO COSMETICS

Short Answer

Place the appropriate key word or short answer in the lines provided.

1. Define a solution. _____

_____

2. Define a solute. _____

_____

3. Define a solvent. _____

_____

4. What is the difference between miscible and immiscible? _____

_____

5. Give an example of a suspension. _____

_____

6. What type of substances are mixed together to form of emulsions?

_____

7. Surfactants have two ends; what are they? _____

_____

Label the Image

8. Under each container (oil-in-water and water-in-oil), list the items that would be examples of these.

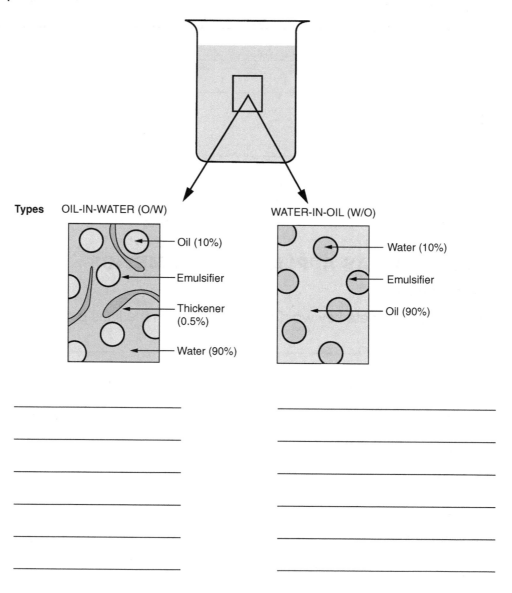

_____   _____

_____   _____

_____   _____

_____   _____

_____   _____

_____   _____

CHEMISTRY REVIEW

Crossword Puzzle

Using the following word bank, place the correct word by the definition and then use it within the crossword puzzle.

oxidation	solute	hydrogen
element	chemistry	lipophilic
molecule	matter	
emulsion	free radicals	

1. _____ Unstable molecules that cause inflammation, disease, and biochemical aging in the body, especially wrinkling and sagging of the skin. They are super oxidizers that cause an oxidation reaction and produce a new one in the process that are created by highly reactive atoms or molecules (often oxygen).

2. _____ A chemical combination of two or more atoms.

3. _____ An unstable mixture of two or more immiscible substances (substances that normally will not stay blended) united with the aid of an emulsifier.

4. _____ Colorless, odorless, tasteless gas; the lightest element known.

5. _____ Either the addition of oxygen or the loss of hydrogen.

6. _____ Any substance that occupies space and has mass (weight).

7. _____ The simplest form of matter; cannot be broken down into a simpler substance without loss of identity.

8. _____ Having an affinity for or an attraction to fat and oils (oil-loving).

9. _____ Science that deals with the composition, structures, and properties of matter and how matter changes under different conditions.

10. _____ A substance that dissolves the solute to form a solution.

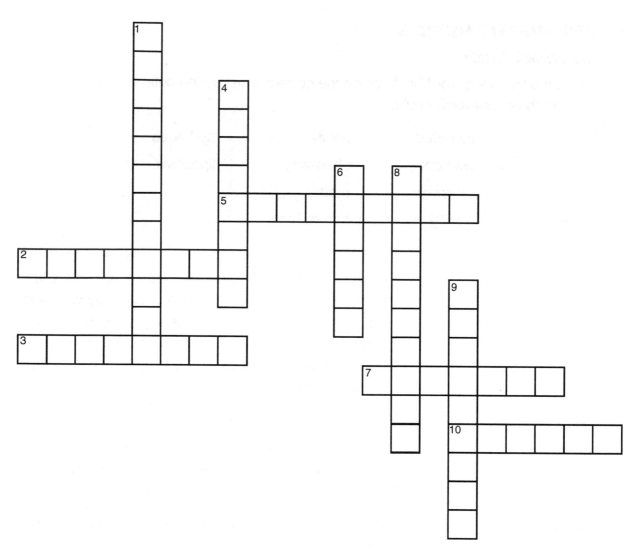

8 Basics of Electricity

Date: _____

Rating: _____

WHY STUDY THE BASICS OF ELECTRICITY?

Short Essay

Why do you feel that you should have a thorough understanding of the basics of electricity? Provide your answer below.

- _____
  _____
  _____

- _____
  _____
  _____

- _____
  _____
  _____

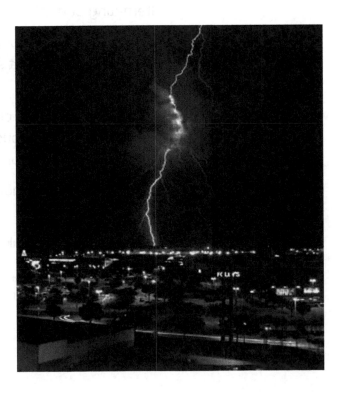

ELECTRICITY REVIEW

Matching

Draw a line from the word to its corresponding definition.

1. Alternating current

the movement of particles around an atom that creates pure energy; form of energy that, when in motion, exhibits magnetic, chemical, or thermal effects

2. Ampere

a special device that prevents excessive current from passing through a circuit

3. Circuit breaker

any substance, material, or medium that easily transmits electricity

4. Complete circuit

known as amp; unit that measures the amount of an electric current

5. Conductor

rapid and interrupted current, flowing first in one direction and then in the opposite direction

6. Converter

the use of electrical devices to treat skin and to provide therapeutic benefits

7. Direct current

switch that automatically interrupts or shuts off an electric circuit

8. Electric current

apparatus that changes direct current to alternating current

9. Electricity

the connection that completes the circuit; also carries the current safely a way to the ground

10. Electrotherapy

the path of an electric current from the generating source through conductors and back to its original source

11. Fuse

substance that does not easily transmit electricity

12. Grounding

the flow of electricity along a conductor

13. Insulator

constant, even-flowing current that travels in one direction only and is produced by chemical means

14. Kilowatt	unit that measures the resistance of an electric current
15. Milliampere	unit that measures the pressure or force that pushes the flow of electrons forward through a conductor
16. Modalities	one-thousandth of an ampere
17. Ohm	measurement of how much electric energy is being used in one second
18. Plug	currents used in electrical facial and scalp treatments
19. Rectifier	1,000 watts
20. Volt	apparatus that changes alternating current to direct current
21. Watt	two- or three-prong connector at the end of an electrical cord that connects an apparatus to an electrical outlet

ELECTROTHERAPY

Fill in the Blank

Fill in the blank with the correct term.

1. Electrical facial treatments are commonly referred to as _____.

2. These treatments are often called _____.

3. An _____ is an applicator for directing the electric current from the device to the client's skin.

4. _____ indicates the negative or positive pole of an electric current.

5. The positive electrode is called an _____.

6. The negative electrode is called a _____.

7. _____ is a constant and direct current (DC). It has a positive and negative pole and produces chemical changes when it passes through the tissues and fluids of the body.

8. _____ is the electrode used on the area to be treated.

9. _____ is the process of introducing water-soluble products into the skin with the use of electric current.

10. _____ refers to infusing a positive (acid) product into the skin.

11. _____ is the process of infusing (alkaline) a negative (alkaline) product into the skin.

12. _____ is a form of anaphoresis and is a process used to soften and emulsify grease deposits (oil) and blackheads in the hair follicles.

MICROCURRENT

Short Answer

List the benefits of microcurrent on the lines below.

- _____
- _____
- _____
- _____
- _____
- _____
- _____
- _____

HIGH FREQUENCY

Short Answer

Answer the following questions in the spaces provided.

1. Describe high frequency.

   _____

   _____

   _____

2. List the benefits of high frequency.

   _____

   _____

   _____

   _____

   _____

3. List the contraindications of high frequency.

_____

_____

_____

_____

_____

_____

_____

_____

_____

_____

_____

_____

Short Essay

4. Explain the difference between direct high frequency application and indirect application.

_____

_____

_____

_____

_____

_____

_____

_____

_____

_____

_____

ELECTROMAGNETIC ENERGY, LASERS, AND LED (LIGHT-EMITTING DIODE)

Fill in the Blank

Answer the following questions in the spaces provided.

1. _____ is the application of light rays to the skin for the treatment of acne, wrinkles, capillaries, pigmentation, or hair removal.

2. _____ is electromagnetic radiation that we can see.

3. A _____ is the distance between the peaks of two successive waves of electromagnetic radiation.

4. Shorter wavelengths have a higher _____ than longer wavelengths.

5. Visible light makes up _____ percent of natural sunlight.

6. Ultraviolet rays and infrared rays are _____ forms of electromagnetic radiation.

7. Among the visible light rays, _____ has the shortest wavelength and _____ has the longest.

8. _____—also called actinic rays—make up _____ percent of natural sunlight.

9. _____ rays cause damage to collagen and fibrils.

10. When compared to visible light, UV rays:

   a) _____

   b) _____

   c) _____

11. _____ are also called the burning rays.

12. Natural sunlight produces Vitamin _____ in the skin.

13. UV rays stimulate the production of _____ in the skin.

14. How many new cases of skin cancer are diagnosed each year? _____ What percentage of cancer cases are caused by overexposure to UV radiation? _____

15. Infrared rays are used in spas and saunas for _____ _____.

16. _____ rays make up 60 percent of natural sunlight.

17. When compared to visible light, infrared rays:

    a) _____

    b) _____

    c) _____

18. _____ light contains few heat rays, is the least penetrating, and has some germicidal and chemical benefits.

19. _____ light is used on dry skin in combination with oils and creams. It produces the most _____ and penetrates the _____.

20. Laser is an acronym for _____.

21. Which device uses multiple colors of focused light to treat spider veins and brown spots? _____

22. _____ devices release a flashing light on the skin that, in turn, releases healing enzymes in the skin that cause healing.

23. LED is the acronym for _____, a medical device used to reduce acne, increase skin circulation, and improve the collagen content in the skin.

24. The LED color of light is also seeking color in the skin known as a _____. This term references a color component within the skin such as blood or melanin.

25. _____ is a light device that uses multiple colors and wavelengths (broad spectrum) of focused light to treat spider veins, hyperpigmentation, rosacea/redness, wrinkles, enlarged hair follicles/pores, and excessive hair.

FACIAL MACHINES

Name the Device

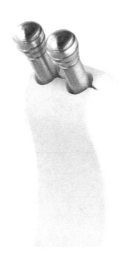

_____

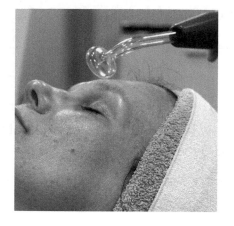

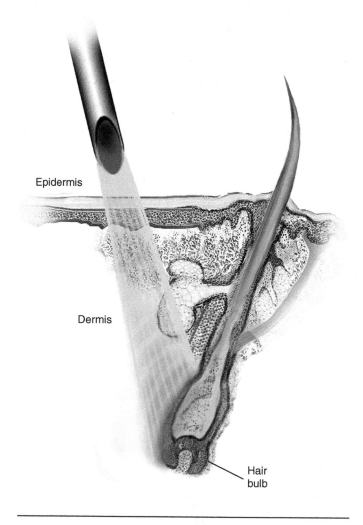

Epidermis

Dermis

Hair
bulb

KEY TERMS

Word Search

Locate the terms from the word bank within the word search.

fuse	conductor	desincrustation	anaphoresis	watt
ampere	laser	electrotherapy	grounding	
polarity	modalities	insulator	ohm	

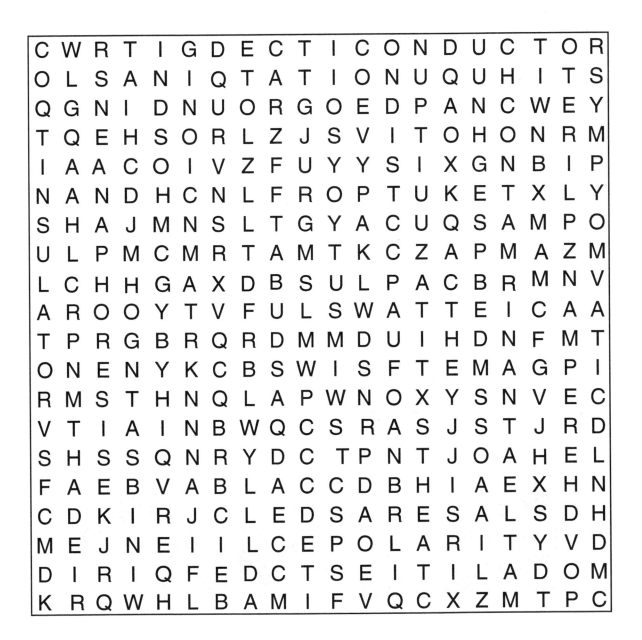

```
C W R T I G D E C T I C O N D U C T O R
O L S A N I Q T A T I O N U Q U H I T S
Q G N I D N U O R G O E D P A N C W E Y
T Q E H S O R L Z J S V I T O H O N R M
I A A C O I V Z F U Y Y S I X G N B I P
N A N D H C N L F R O P T U K E T X L Y
S H A J M N S L T G Y A C U Q S A M P O
U L P M C M R T A M T K C Z A P M A Z M
L C H H G A X D B S U L P A C B R M N V
A R O O Y T V F U L S W A T T E I C A A
T P R G B R Q R D M M D U I H D N F M T
O N E N Y K C B S W I S F T E M A G P I
R M S T H N Q L A P W N O X Y S N V E C
V T I A I N B W Q C S R A S J S T J R D
S H S S Q N R Y D C T P N T J O A H E L
F A E B V A B L A C C D B H I A E X H N
C D K I R J C L E D S A R E S A L S D H
M E J N E I I L C E P O L A R I T Y V D
D I R I Q F E D C T S E I T I L A D O M
K R Q W H L B A M I F V Q C X Z M T P C
```

CHAPTER 9 Basics of Nutrition

Date: _____

Rating: _____

WHY STUDY NUTRITION?

Short Essay

On the lines below, explain why it is important to learn about nutrition.

_____

_____

_____

_____

_____

_____

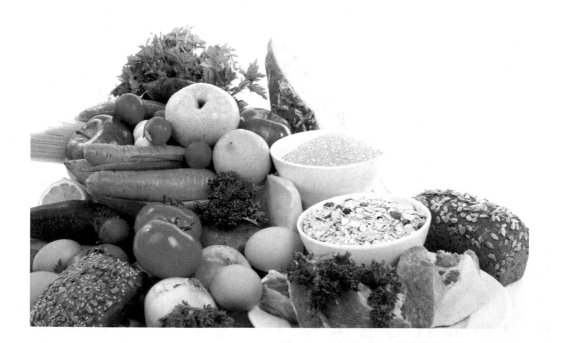

NUTRITIOUS DIET

Mind Mapping

Mind mapping creates a free-flowing outline of material or information. Using the central or key point of *nutrition*, map out what nutrition means to you and how you can have a nutritious diet. Use terms, pictures, and symbols as desired. Using color will increase memory of the material.

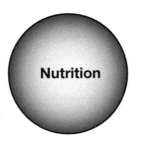

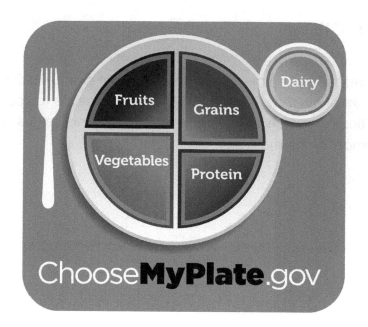

ChooseMyPlate.gov

© USDA.

NUTRIENTS

Word Scramble

Unscramble the following terms using the definitions as clues.

TSFA	_____	Also known as lipids.
ANMIO DCAIS	_____	Proteins contain these.
ZYEMSEN	_____	Biological catalysts.
CRMUTTSNANOREI	_____	Nutrients that make up the largest part of nutrition.
RETNNIOTI	_____	Used in the treatment of acne.
FLBONODSIAVOI	_____	Also known as Vitamin P.
LORIECSA	_____	A measure of heat units from food.
RLSINMEA	_____	These are required for many reactions of the cells.
ROHDYAECBRTESA	_____	Compounds that break down the basic chemical sugars and supply the body with energy.
RECSSIAOLREOT	_____	Hardening of the arteries.
GLHYIAOPCYME	_____	A condition when blood sugar drops too low.

DIET ESSENTIALS

Word Search

Find the answers to the following clues in the word search.

1. _____ LDLs and HDLs are in this category.

2. _____ Inorganic materials that are essential in many cells.

3. _____ An example of this would be glucose.

4. Nutrients are broken down into _____ triphosphate.

5. _____ Too much of these in the diet can lead to obesity.

6. _____ This is when a vitamin has been added to a food product.

7. _____ This is a catalyst that breaks down food.

8. _____ A polyunsaturated fat necessary for brain development.

9. _____ Is a chain of amino acids used in cell functions for body growth.

10. _____ An antioxidant that helps protect the skin.

```
A N I E T O R P C U F C T O R W U B H P
C X F S S I O N S T A F E M E N T I T S
J W O I D N S O R G W Q P V Q M B C S Q
L O P I O M E G A T T A I C Y R P B R G
M B Q C O I V Z T P Y T P N Z R N B N E
G C R D L O P R F W A V O U K E S I L N
I H W J M Y S P T M H I C U C S E M P Z
P O Z M C I R Q I G S K C A A T N A E Y
D L J H F I X N B L U P R A E B I M R M
X E S O Y C E F A L Q B W S M E S C F E
B S D H C S Q R D M O D L I H Z O F E S
Q T F O Y T E B S H I A F T I M N G C I
S E R U H N Q L Y P O N P T C S E V T C
M R J B I N B D Q G V S I R J S D J G D
B O Q M Q N R Y D C T R N T J V A H O L
W L B C V A S L A C V D B H I A E F N N
X Z L T T J C L E I S A E T S Y P T D H
D B J E E I G L R E P O L A R I T Y V D
R Y S O Q F Q P D E I F I T R O F V O Q
S O W T J M C B N V F V W C Y Z Q W P V
```

PROTEINS

Fill in the Blank

Finish the sentences using a word from the word list below.

deoxyribonucleic acid	anemia
complementary	legumes
elastin	amino acids
macronutrients	poultry
nonessential	antibodies

1. _____ are the basic building blocks necessary for bodily functions, including the skin.

2. Proteins are chains of _____, molecules that are used by every cell of the body.

3. Proteins are used in the duplication of _____.

4. Collagen and _____ are made from protein.

5. Eleven of the 20 common amino acids are called _____ amino acids.

6. Proteins are used by the immune system in making _____.

7. Good sources of proteins are eggs, dairy products, fish, and _____.

8. _____ foods are two incomplete sources of proteins.

9. Vegetarians can consume proteins from nuts, grains, vegetables, and _____.

10. A deficiency in protein can lead to _____.

CARBOHYDRATES

Fill in the Blank

Finish the sentences using a word from the word list below.

sugars	mucopolysaccharides
monosaccharides	fiber
glucose	simple
adenosine triphosphate	insoluble
apples	oxygen

1. Carbohydrates break down the basic chemical _____ that supply energy for the body.

2. The substance that provides energy to cells is called _____.

3. ATP converts _____ into carbon dioxide.

4. _____ are carbohydrate–lipid complexes that are good water binders.

5. A good example of a basic unit of a carbohydrate is glucose, which is known as a _____.

6. The three basic types of carbohydrates are simple sugars, starches, and _____.

7. There are two categories of carbohydrates that help move food particles through the digestive tract—soluble and _____.

8. Fruits and vegetables have both _____ sugars and fiber.

9. _____ can drop too low without adequate carbohydrates.

10. High fiber foods include grains, brans, beans, and _____.

FATS

Fill in the Blank

saturated	omega-3 fatty acids
salmon	triglycerides
energy	hormones
linoleic acid	lipids
hardening	carbohydrates

Finish the sentences using a word from the word list above.

1. Fats are used as _____, but not as readily as carbohydrates.

2. Fats are also called _____.

3. Fats in the body make _____ as well as create cell membranes.

4. Ninety-five percent of fat intake comes from _____.

5. Processed foods have _____ fats.

6. The type of fats that have more rigid molecules can cause _____ of the arteries.

7. Fats can be made from the body from _____ and proteins.

8. A "good" polyunsaturated fat that may decrease the clogging of the arteries is called _____.

9. The "good" polyunsaturated fat can be found in tuna, trout, and _____.

10. _____ helps create the lipid barrier of the skin.

FOOD GROUPS

Label the Image

Label each picture with carbohydrates, fats, or proteins. Some may have more than one answer.

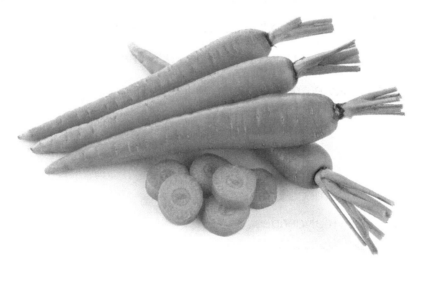

© atoss, 2011/www.shutterstock.com.

_____

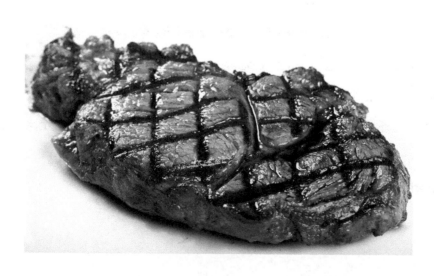

© Dan Peretz, 2011/www.shutterstock.com.

_____

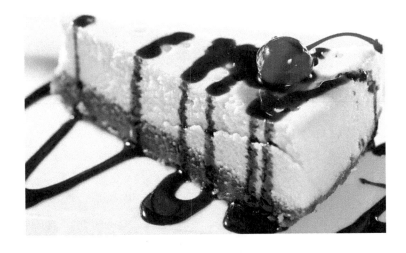

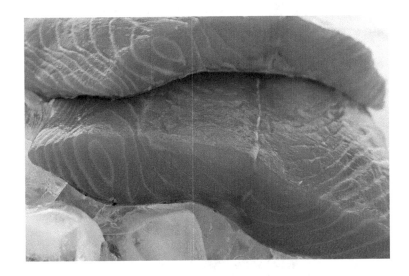

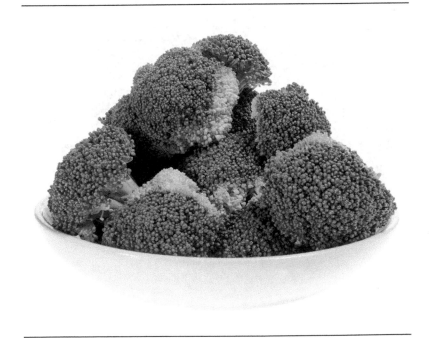

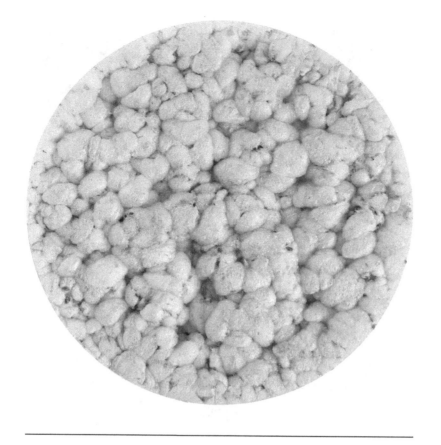

_____

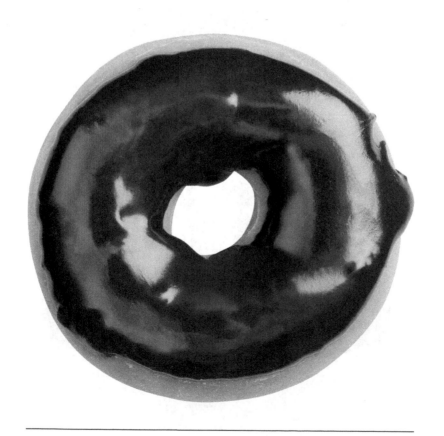

_____

VITAMINS AND MINERALS

Matching

Match the vitamin or mineral with its source and its function.

A	inositol	K	manganese
B-1	B-complex (niacin)	P	phosphorus
B-2	B-complex (PABA)	calcium	potassium
B-6	B-15	chromium	sodium
B-7	C	copper	sulphur
B-12	D	iodine	zinc
choline	E	iron	selenium
folic acid	F	magnesium	fluoride

SOURCE: Grains, nuts, fish, poultry, wheat germ, legumes, meat

FUNCTION: Metabolism, appetite maintenance, nerve function, healthy mental state

VITAMIN/MINERAL: _____

SOURCE: Table salt, shellfish, meat, poultry

FUNCTION: Maintains muscular, blood, and lymph systems

VITAMIN/MINERAL: _____

SOURCE: Egg yolks, organ meats, fish, fortified milk

FUNCTION: Healthy bone formation, healthy circulatory functions, nervous system

VITAMIN/MINERAL: _____

SOURCE: Lecithin, fish, wheat germ, egg yolk, soybeans

FUNCTION: Nerve metabolism and transmission; regulates liver, kidneys, and gall bladder

VITAMIN/MINERAL: _____

SOURCE: Yellow and green fruits and vegetables, carrots, dairy products, fish, liver oil

FUNCTION: Growth and repair of body tissues, bone formation, vision

VITAMIN/MINERAL: _____

SOURCE: Grains, vegetables, bananas, legumes

FUNCTION: Fluid balance; controls activity of heart muscle, nervous system, and kidneys

VITAMIN/MINERAL: _____

SOURCE: Water, toothpaste

FUNCTION: Bone and teeth formation

VITAMIN/MINERAL: _____

SOURCE: Whole grains, green, leafy vegetables, liver, fish, eggs

FUNCTION: Metabolism, health in hair, skin, and nails, cell respiration, formation of antibodies and red blood cells

VITAMIN/MINERAL: _____

SOURCE: Whole grains, wheat bran

FUNCTION: Healthy digestion and metabolism, reproductive system, aids in healing

VITAMIN/MINERAL: _____

SOURCE: Whole grains, green, leafy vegetables, yeast, bananas, organ meats

FUNCTION: Formation of antibodies, sodium/potassium balance

VITAMIN/MINERAL: _____

SOURCE: Whole grain, citrus fruits, yeast, molasses, milk

FUNCTION: Hair growth, metabolism, lecithin formation

VITAMIN/MINERAL: _____

SOURCE: Whole grains, pumpkin and sesame seeds

FUNCTION: Metabolism, stimulates nerve and glandular system, cellular respiration

VITAMIN/MINERAL: _____

SOURCE: Eggs, milk/milk products, fish, organ meats

FUNCTION: Metabolism, healthy nervous system, blood cell formation

VITAMIN/MINERAL: _____

SOURCE: Green, leafy vegetables, organ meats, yeast, milk products

FUNCTION: Red blood cell formation, growth, and division

VITAMIN/MINERAL: _____

SOURCE: Green, leafy vegetables, milk, kelp, safflower oil

FUNCTION: Blood clotting agent, important to proper liver function and
                           longevity

VITAMIN/MINERAL: _____

SOURCE: Green vegetables, wheat germ, organ meats, eggs,
                           vegetable oils

FUNCTION: Red blood cells, inhibits coagulation of blood, cellular
                           respiration

VITAMIN/MINERAL: _____

SOURCE: Meats, fish, green, leafy vegetables

FUNCTION: Hemoglobin formation, blood quality, resistance to stress
                           and disease

VITAMIN/MINERAL: _____

SOURCE: Citrus fruits, vegetables, tomatoes, potatoes

FUNCTION: Aids in healing, collagen maintenance, resistance to
                           disease

VITAMIN/MINERAL: _____

SOURCE: Iodized table salt, shellfish

FUNCTION: Part of the hormone thyroxine, which controls metabolism

VITAMIN/MINERAL: _____

SOURCE: Meat, poultry, fish, milk   products, peanuts

FUNCTION: Metabolism; healthy skin, tongue, and digestive system;
                           blood circulation; essential for synthesis of sex hormones

VITAMIN/MINERAL: _____

SOURCE: Fruits

FUNCTION: For healthy connective tissue, aids in utilization of Vitamin C

VITAMIN/MINERAL: _____

SOURCE: Fish, eggs, nuts, cabbage, meat

FUNCTION: Collagen and body tissue formation, gives strength to keratin

VITAMIN/MINERAL: _____

SOURCE: Dairy products, bone meal

FUNCTION: Resilient bones, teeth, muscle tissue; regulates heartbeat;
                           blood clotting

VITAMIN/MINERAL: _____

SOURCE: Corn oil, yeast, clams, whole grains

FUNCTION: Body's use of glucose, energy, effective use of insulin

VITAMIN/MINERAL: _____

SOURCE: Nuts, green vegetables, whole grains

FUNCTION: Metabolism

VITAMIN/MINERAL: _____

SOURCE: Egg yolks, legumes, whole grains

FUNCTION: Carbohydrate and fat production, sex hormone production, bone development

VITAMIN/MINERAL: _____

SOURCE: Wheat germ, seeds, vegetable oils

FUNCTION: Respiration of body organs, lubrication of cells, blood coagulation, glandular activity

VITAMIN/MINERAL: _____

SOURCE: Whole grains, green, leafy vegetables, seafood, almonds

FUNCTION: Healthy red blood cells, bone growth and formation, joins with Vitamin C to form elastin

VITAMIN/MINERAL: _____

SOURCE: Whole grains, liver, meat, fish

FUNCTION: Part of important antioxidant, glutathione peroxidase

VITAMIN/MINERAL: _____

SOURCE: Proteins, grains

FUNCTION: Bone development, important in protein, fat and carbohydrate utilization

VITAMIN/MINERAL: _____

CRITICAL THINKING

Short Essay

1. In your own words, explain the difference between fats, fatty acids, and trans-fatty acids. What are the benefits? What are the negative components?

_____

_____

_____

_____

_____

_____

_____

_____

_____

_____

_____

_____

_____

_____

2. Research other fatty components such as fatty alcohols and explain where they can be found and what do they do.

_____

_____

_____

_____

VITAMINS AND MINERALS

Matching

Draw a line from the vitamin to the importance of it.

Bioflavanoids	Promotes wound healing and helps the immune system.
Vitamin C	Helps prevent osteoporosis.
Pyridoxine	Also known as the sunshine vitamin.
Vitamin D	Helps in collagen formation.
Riboflavin	It is needed for the proper repair of the skin and tissues.
Vitamin A	Deficiencies can result in cheilosis.
Copper	Protects capillary blood vessels.
Calcium	Also known as retinol and will help with exfoliation.
Zinc	It is important in the metabolism of proteins.

WEIGHT LOSS

Short Answer

List the seven truths about weight loss below.

1. _____

_____

_____

2. _____

_____

_____

3. _____

_____

_____

4. _____

_____

_____

5. _____

_____

_____

6. _____

_____

_____

7. _____

_____

_____

WATER

Short Answer

1. Water has many, many benefits. List at least five benefits of water below.

_____

_____

_____

_____

_____

_____

2. Write below how many ounces you have been drinking for the past 3 days.

How much water do you drink daily?

Day One: Morning water intake: _____ ounces of water

Afternoon water intake: _____ ounces of water

Evening water intake: _____ ounces of water

Total daily intake: _____ ounces of water

Should be at least 72–96 ounces of water.

Day Two: Morning water intake: _____ ounces of water

Afternoon water intake: _____ ounces of water

Evening water intake: _____ ounces of water

Total daily intake: _____ ounces of water

Should be at least 72–96 ounces of water.

Day Three: Morning water intake: _____ ounces of water

Afternoon water intake: _____ ounces of water

Evening water intake: _____ ounces of water

Total daily intake: _____ ounces of water

Should be at least 72–96 ounces of water.

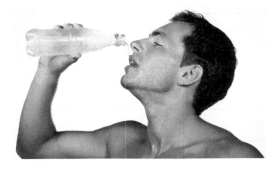

NUTRITION RECOMMENDATIONS

Short Essay

In order to maintain a healthy lifestyle, making healthy choices for your food intake should be a main priority. As we go through our daily lives, we may not always make the healthiest choices when it comes to eating. Referring to the *MyPlate* featured on page 201 in your textbook: What are some ways you can incorporate the suggestions into your diet? Based on *MyPlate*, what are some areas of your diet that need improvement? What steps do you plan on taking to make your diet healthier and more sustainable? In an essay, explain some of the changes you plan on making to your diet and why.

_____

_____

_____

_____

_____

_____

_____

_____

_____

_____

_____

_____

_____

_____

_____

_____

_____

_____

_____

NUTRITION FACTS

True/False

Determine if the following statements are true or false.

T   F   **1.** The letters *DASH* in DASH diet stand for Dietary Approaches to Staying Healthy.

T   F   **2.** Macronutrients are the three basic food groups.

T   F   **3.** Lactose and sucrose are examples of carbohydrates.

T   F   **4.** Fiber is an example of protein.

T   F   **5.** Hypoglycemia is when you have low blood sugar.

T   F   **6.** The main lipid in the cell membranes is insulin.

T   F   **7.** Examples of fat-soluble vitamins would be B and C.

T   F   **8.** Calories are a measure of heat units.

T   F   **9.** Micronutrients are the vitamins and minerals found in foods.

T   F   **10.** Enzymes are known as biological amino acids.

T   F   **11.** Vitamin E is also known as tocopherol.

T   F   **12.** Osteoporosis is a reduction in the quality of bone.

T   F   **13.** Niacin is a vitamin that falls into the Vitamin C category.

T   F   **14.** Vitamin K helps the blood coagulate.

T   F   **15.** Folacin falls into the Vitamin B category.

T   F   **16.** Bioflavanoids are also referred to as Vitamin C.

T   F   **17.** Sodium helps regulate the pH of the blood.

T   F   **18.** You must eat a balanced diet for vitamins to have an effect on your body.

T   F   **19.** Water composes 50 to 70 percent of the body's weight.

T   F   **20.** A fad diet may be accompanied by exaggerated claims or promises.

10 Physiology and Histology of the Skin

Date: _____

Rating: _____

WHY STUDY PHYSIOLOGY AND HISTOLOGY OF THE SKIN?

Short Essay

Why do you think estheticians should have a thorough understanding of the physiology and histology of the skin? Provide your answer on the lines below.

_____

_____

_____

_____

_____

_____

_____

_____

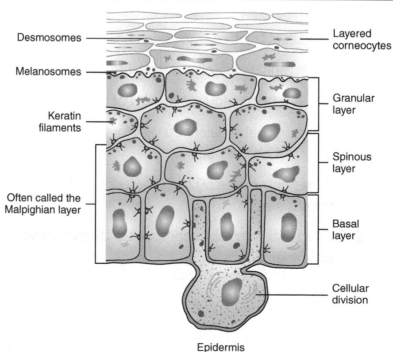

Desmosomes

Melanosomes

Keratin filaments

Often called the Malpighian layer

Layered corneocytes

Granular layer

Spinous layer

Basal layer

Cellular division

Epidermis

© Milady, a part of Cengage Learning.

SKIN FACTS

Fill in the Blank

On the spaces below, list as many skin facts as you can. The first three are filled in for you.

1. Skin, or the integumentary system, is the largest organ in the body.

2. It is a strong barrier designed to protect us from the outside elements.

3. Hormones, growth factors, and other biochemicals control the skin's intricate functions.

4. _____

_____

5. _____

_____

6. _____

_____

7. _____

_____

8. _____

_____

PROTECTION

Define the Term

Define the following terms.

1. acid mantle: _____

_____

_____

2. barrier function: _____

_____

_____

_____

_____

_____

_____

3. transepidermal water loss (TEWL): _____

_____

4. epidermal growth factor: _____

_____

_____

5. fibroblasts: _____

_____

_____

SKIN PROTECTION

Short Answer

Put the correct answer for the following questions on the lines provided below.

1. What is the pH of the skin? _____

2. How does melanin protect the skin? _____

_____

3. How does the body protect itself from extreme temperature? _____

_____

_____

_____

4. How does the body maintain thermoregulation? _____

_____

5. How do the arrector pili muscles aid in thermoregulation? _____

_____

_____

_____

6. What glands are used by the body to excrete salt, water, and unwanted chemicals? _____

7. What glands are used by the body to rid the skin of excess oil? _____

_____

8. What exactly is secreted by the sebaceous glands? _____

9. What would be the reason a product could get absorbed into the body?

_____

LAYERS OF THE SKIN

Matching

Match the following terms with their descriptions below.

stratum corneum	melanin	arrector pili
dermis	adipose	elastin
epidermis	collagen	hyaluronic acid
keratin	sebaceous	tactile

_____ **1.** refers to the substance that keeps skin soft and protected

_____ **2.** deeper layer of the skin

_____ **3.** fiber protein that provides resiliency and protection to the skin

_____ **4.** top layer of the skin

_____ **5.** outermost layer of the skin

_____ **6.** skin pigment

_____ **7.** muscles that cause goose bumps

_____ **8.** a glycosaminoglycan (GAG) that hydrates the skin

_____ **9.** sense of touch

_____ **10.** subcutaneous layer composed of fat

_____ **11.** makes up 70 percent of the dermis

_____ **12.** fibrous protein that forms elastic tissue and gives skin its elasticity

STRUCTURE OF THE SKIN

Label the Image

From the following list of parts of the skin, identify the numbered parts on the illustration. Insert the proper term in the space provided.

adipose (fatty) tissue	mouth of follicle	stratum granulosum
arrector pili muscle	papillary layer of dermis	stratum lucidum
arteries	reticular layer of dermis	stratum spinosum
dermal papilla	sebaceous (oil) gland	subcutaneous tissue
dermis (true skin)	stratum corneum	sudoriferous gland
epidermis	stratum germinativum	sweat pore
hair shaft	(basal layer)	veins

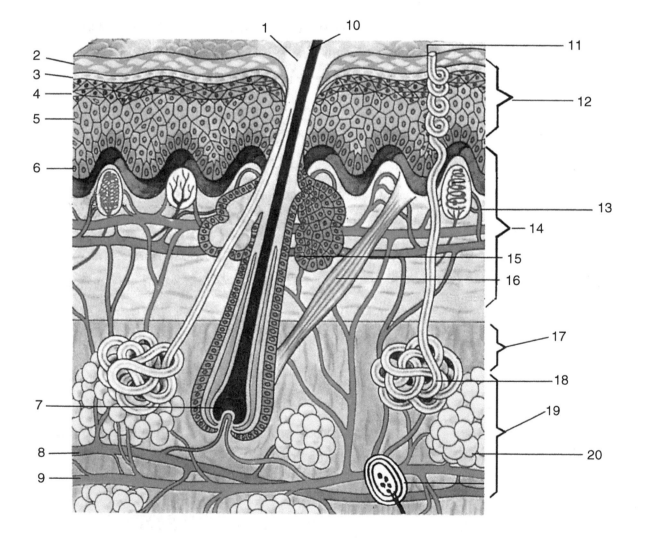

© Milady, a part of Cengage Learning.

1. _____

2. _____

3. _____

4. _____

5. _____

6. _____

7. _____

8. _____

9. _____

10. _____

11. _____

12. _____

13. _____

14. _____

15. _____

16. _____

17. _____

18. _____

19. _____

20. _____

LAYERS OF THE SKIN

Short Answer

In the space below, list the layers of the epidermis

_____

_____

_____

_____

_____

SKIN COLOR: MELANIN, MELANOCYTES, AND MELANOSOMES

Fill in the Blank

Choose the word from the word bank that best fits the description.

melanin	tyrosinase inhibitors
tyrosinase	dendrite
eumelanin	pheomelanin
melanocyte	

_____ **1.** It is the pigment that protects us from the sun.

_____ **2.** This is the cell that creates the melanosome sphere.

_____ **3.** This is the route that is taken when a melanocyte will deposit pigment-carrying melanosomes into about 30 keratinocytes.

_____ **4.** This is the enzyme that stimulates melanocytes and thus produces melanin.

_____ **5.** This is the pigment that is red to yellow in color.

_____ **6.** This is the pigment that is dark brown to black.

_____ **7.** These are also called brightening agents and can lighten the skin.

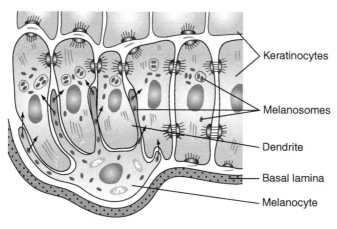

Keratinocytes

Melanosomes

Dendrite

Basal lamina

Melanocyte

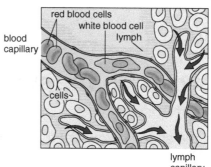

red blood cells
white blood cell
lymph
blood capillary
cells
lymph capillary

OVERVIEW

Word Search

Answer the following questions and then find the word within the word search.

1. What is the technical name for a nail? _____

2. Hair is an example of which type of keratin? _____

3. Motor nerves, such as ones that stimulate the arrector pili muscles, are also known as which type of nerve? _____

4. Sensory nerves, such as ones that feel cold and heat, are also known as which type of nerve? _____

5. Which type of sudoriferous gland is found under the arms? _____

6. Which type of sudoriferous gland is found all over the body? _____

7. What are the two ways that the skin is nourished? _____ and _____

8. UVA rays are known as which type of ray? _____

9. UVB rays are known as which type of ray? _____

10. What is the binding of a protein molecule to a glucose molecule resulting in the formation of damaged, nonfunctioning structures, known as advanced glycation end products, called? _____

11. What is the name of the chronic vascular disorder where telangiectasia is visible? _____

```
Q X S D I G D E C T I D P A B D O O L B
P M R A N I Q T P T I O T V Q U P I S S
R A O I A P O C R I N E D K A T Q O B Y
H R F H S O R L T J S V N U D H E N P M
S A B C O I V P D U Y O S K X G C B J P
A B O D N C O V Y R I P T A K E C X M Y
F I B J Y R Q L T T Y A G U Q S R V P O
F M Q M X N U T A M T I C Z A P I A Z C
E D I I G A I C B S N L P A Q B N M N V
R S P O Y T Y F U G S W A T A E E C A Q
E P S F B L T R I M M E U I H D N F P T
N O F N G K D B T A I S G T E M V G T I
T N T U H C Q L E P W N O X Y B N V N C
W U J B I P I C Q C S R A S J U C J E D
T I T T Q N A Y I C T P N H J R A H R L
G B F C V S R L R C C D P H I N Z Y E N
H E L R O J D L E D S M R E S I L S F H
I F K R E I J L D E Y O L A R N V Q F D
E J S J Q F F D C L S E I T I G N D E M
M A X T F L C A M I F V Q C X Q O U E P
```

CHAPTER 11 Disorders and Diseases of the Skin

Date: _____

Rating: _____

WHY STUDY DISORDERS AND DISEASES OF THE SKIN?

Short Essay

On the lines below, write the reason why you think that estheticians should study and have a thorough understanding of disorders and diseases of the skin?

_____

_____

_____

_____

_____

DISEASES

Mind Mapping

Around the word *diseases*, write as many diseases as you can think of.

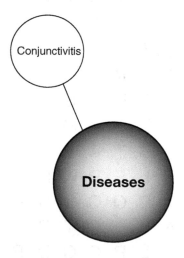

© Milady, a part of Cengage Learning.

DISORDERS

Mind Mapping

Around the word *disorders*, write as many disorders as you can think of.

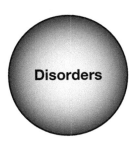

Disorders

DERMATOLOGY AND ESTHETICS

Label the Image

Being able to recognize various skin diseases and disorders is an important part of an esthetician's job. Even though you should never diagnose a client, it is helpful to know which lesions you should and should not work on.

Label the following primary lesions.

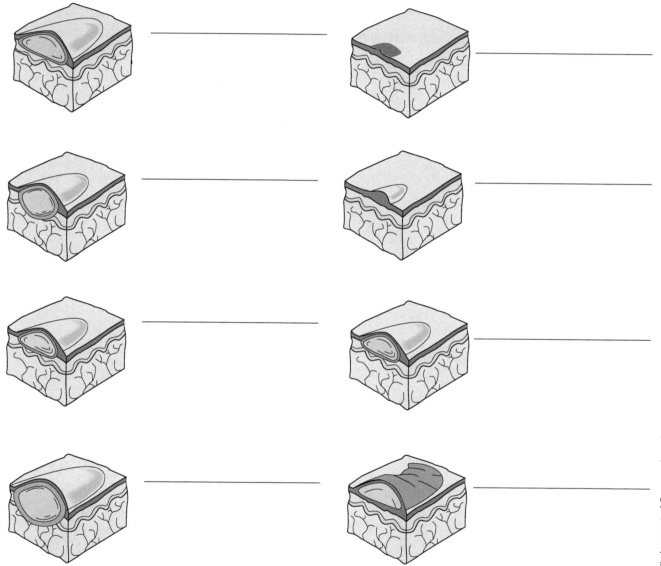

Label the following secondary lesions.

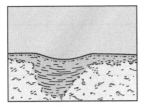 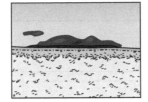 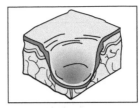

_____ _____ _____

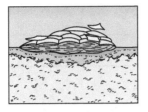 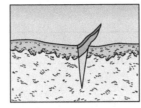 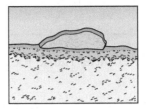

_____ _____ _____

DISORDERS OF THE SEBACEOUS (OIL) GLANDS

Short Answer

Answer the following questions in the spaces provided.

1. Describe acne. _____

   _____

   _____

   _____

   _____

2. What is the name of a disorder that is characterized by dry, scaly skin from sebum deficiency? _____

3. What is a comedone? _____

   _____

4. What is another name for a boil? _____

5. What is a group of boils called? _____

6. What do milia look like? _____

   _____

   _____

7. Describe sebaceous hyperplasia. _____

_____

_____

_____

8. What is caused by severe oiliness of the skin as in an abnormal secretion from the sebaceous glands? _____

9. Describe seborrheic dermatitis. _____

_____

10. What is another name for a steatoma? _____

DISORDERS OF THE SUDORIFEROUS (SWEAT) GLANDS

Short Answer

Answer the following questions in the spaces provided.

1. What is a deficiency in perspiration due to failure of the sweat glands that often results from a fever or skin disease called? _____

2. Describe bromidrosis. _____

_____

3. What is excessive perspiration called? _____

4. What is the technical name for prickly heat? _____

INFLAMMATIONS OF THE SKIN

Short Answer

Answer the following questions in the spaces provided.

1. Explain how dermatitis appears on the skin. _____

_____

2. What causes atopic dermatitis and what type of irritation does it cause?

_____

3. Describe contact dermatitis. _____

_____

_____

_____

4. How is perioral dermatitis different from the other types of dermatitis?

_____

5. Describe eczema. _____

_____

6. What do you call swelling from a fluid imbalance in the cells or from a response to injury, infection, or medication? _____

7. Describe erythema. _____

8. What is the difference between folliculitis and pseudofolliculitis? _____

_____

_____

9. What is the medical term for itching? _____

10. Describe psoriasis. _____

_____

_____

11. What is the technical term for hives? _____

VASCULAR LESIONS

Short Answer

Answer the following questions in the spaces provided.

1. Define rosacea. _____

_____

_____

_____

2. What can aggravate rosacea? _____

_____

3. Define telangiectasia. _____

_____

4. How can varicose veins be treated? _____

HYPERPIGMENTATION AND HYPOPIGMENTATION DISORDERS

Short Answer

Answer the following questions in the spaces provided.

1. Define chloasma. _____

_____

_____

2. Define hyperpigmentation. _____

_____

_____

3. What is the technical term for freckle? _____

4. At what point in someone's life could melasma present itself? _____

_____

5. What is another name for birthmark? _____

6. What is the difference between a stain and a port wine stain? _____

_____

7. Define albinism. _____

_____

_____

_____

8. Define leukoderma. _____

_____

_____

_____

9. Define vitiligo. _____

_____

_____

_____

HYPERTROPHIES

Matching

Match the terms with the correct photograph.

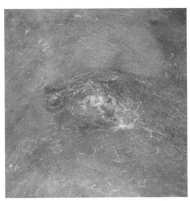

keratosis pilaris

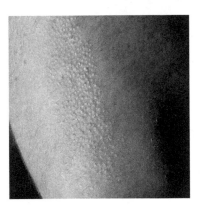

skin tag

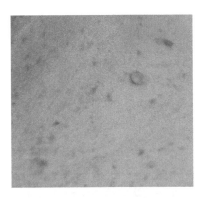

verruca

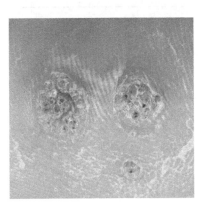

actinic keratosis

CONTAGIOUS AND NON-CONTAGIOUS DISEASES

Fill in the Blanks

Fill in the correct medical term on the lines provided.

1. wart _____

2. pinkeye _____

3. fungal infection _____

4. shingles _____

5. fever blisters _____

6. impetigo _____

7. tinea versicolor _____

8. genital herpes _____

9. ringworm _____

SKIN CANCER

Under each photograph, list at least three facts for each type of skin cancer.

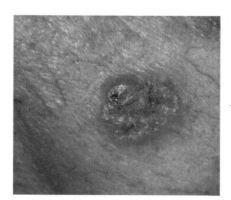

Basal cell carcinoma

1. _____

_____

2. _____

_____

3. _____

_____

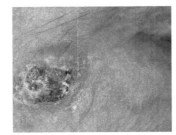

Squamous cell
carcinoma

1. _____

_____

2. _____

_____

3. _____

_____

Malignant
melanoma

1. _____

_____

_____

2. _____

_____

_____

3. _____

_____

_____

_____

_____

_____

_____

_____

_____

_____

MELANOMA

Fill in the Blank

Explain what the letters stand for in the ABCDEs of melanoma.

A _____

_____

B _____

_____

C _____

_____

D _____

_____

E _____

_____

ACNE

Short Answer

Acne is a primary concern for many clients seeking skin care help from an esthetician. This severe skin problem can greatly affect a person's self-esteem. Acne, a skin disorder of the sebaceous glands, is characterized by comedones and blemishes and is hereditary. It is usually triggered by hormonal changes. It begins to flare up when a person reaches puberty, but adult acne is also prevalent.

Answer the following questions.

1. What are the causes of acne? _____

_____

_____

2. Describe retention hyperkeratosis. _____

_____

_____

3. What is the name of the bacteria that causes acne? _____

4. What do papules look like? _____

5. What is the name of the male hormone that triggers acne? _____

6. What does comedogenic mean? _____

7. What is the technical name for breakouts caused by rubbing or touching the face? _____

On the following spaces, describe the four types of acne.

8. Grade I _____

_____

_____

_____

9. Grade II _____

_____

_____

_____

10. Grade III _____

_____

_____

_____

11. Grade IV _____

_____

_____

_____

SKIN DISORDERS AND DISEASES

Word Search

Find the following words from the word bank within the word search.

wheal	tinea	urticaria
asteatosis	hyperpigmentation	mole
carbuncle	leukoderma	scale
pustule	psoriasis	bulla
tan		

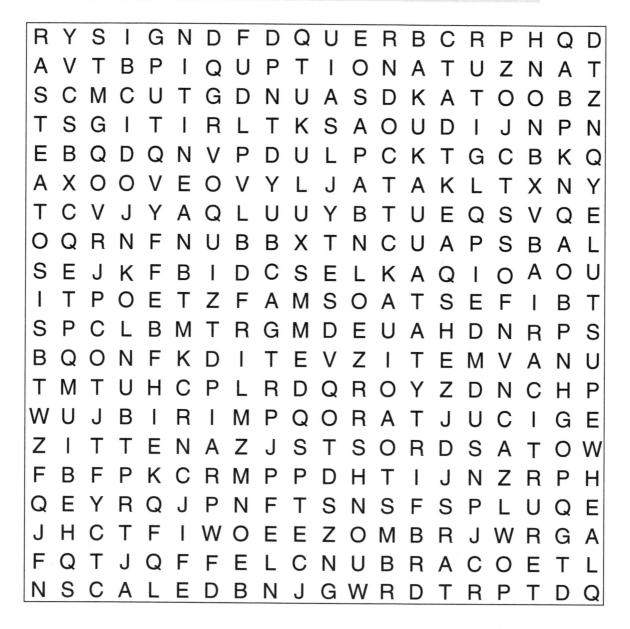

```
R Y S I G N D F D Q U E R B C R P H Q D
A V T B P I Q U P T I O N A T U Z N A T
S C M C U T G D N U A S D K A T O O B Z
T S G I T I R L T K S A O U D I J N P N
E B Q D Q N V P D U L P C K T G C B K Q
A X O O V E O V Y L J A T A K L T X N Y
T C V J Y A Q L U U Y B T U E Q S V Q E
O Q R N F N U B B X T N C U A P S B A L
S E J K F B I D C S E L K A Q I O A O U
I T P O E T Z F A M S O A T S E F I B T
S P C L B M T R G M D E U A H D N R P S
B Q O N F K D I T E V Z I T E M V A N U
T M T U H C P L R D Q R O Y Z D N C H P
W U J B I R I M P Q O R A T J U C I G E
Z I T T E N A Z J S T S O R D S A T O W
F B F P K C R M P P D H T I J N Z R P H
Q E Y R Q J P N F T S N S F S P L U Q E
J H C T F I W O E E Z O M B R J W R G A
F Q T J Q F F E L C N U B R A C O E T L
N S C A L E D B N J G W R D T R P T D Q
```

12 Skin Analysis

Date: _____

Rating: _____

WHY STUDY SKIN ANALYSIS?

Short Essay

What are some of the reasons that estheticians should have a thorough understanding of skin analysis? Provide your answer below.

_____

_____

_____

_____

_____

_____

_____

_____

_____

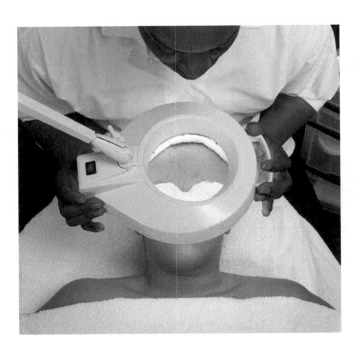

SKIN TYPES ARE GENETICALLY DETERMINED

Short Essay

In your own words, describe each of the skin types and what would be beneficial to each type.

1. DRY SKIN:

_____

_____

_____

WHAT WOULD BENEFIT DRY SKIN:

_____

_____

_____

2. DEHYDRATED SKIN:

_____

_____

_____

WHAT WOULD BENEFIT DEHYDRATED SKIN:

_____

_____

_____

3. NORMAL SKIN:

_____

_____

_____

WHAT WOULD BENEFIT NORMAL SKIN:

_____

_____

_____

4. COMBINATION SKIN:

_____

_____

_____

WHAT WOULD BENEFIT COMBINATION SKIN:

_____

_____

_____

5. OILY SKIN:

_____

_____

_____

WHAT WOULD BENEFIT OILY SKIN:

_____

_____

_____

6. SENSITIVE SKIN:

_____

_____

_____

WHAT WOULD BENEFIT SENSITIVE SKIN:

_____

_____

_____

THE FITZPATRICK SCALE

Fill in the Chart

The Fitzpatrick Scale is a common scale used to measure the skin type's ability to tolerate sun exposure. Fill in the missing sections of the chart.

Fitzpatrick Skin General Characteristics	Type	Appearance and Skin Reaction to the Sun	Risk
	I	Very fair; blond or red hair; light-colored eyes; freckles common. Always burns, never tans.	High risk for skin cancer, vascular damage.
	II	Fair-skinned; light eyes; light hair. Burns easily, tans with difficulty.	
	III		
	IV		High risk of hyper/hypopigmentation. High risk for scarring. Moderate risk for vascular damage

Fitzpatrick Skin General Characteristics	Type	Appearance and Skin Reaction to the Sun	Risk
	V		
	VI	Black skin, brown eyes; rarely sun sensitive. Tans easily; may never burn.	

DIVERSE SKIN PIGMENTATION

Fill in the Blank

Fill in the blanks with the correct answers from the word bank below.

thicker	melanin	hyperpigmentation
Asian skin	post-inflamatory hyperpigmentaton	keloids
melanosome		

1. Darker skin types contain more _____ than lighter Caucasian skin types do.

2. The number of melanocytes is the same, but the melanin transferred to keratinocytes by the _____ is greater in dark skin.

3. _____ is a greater problem for darker skin types.

4. _____ can result from hormones, trauma, extractions, sun damage, or exfoliation.

5. Abnormal hypertrophic scarring, also known as _____, is also problematic for black skin.

6. _____ is considered to be one of the most sensitive skin types.

7. Native American, Indian, and Hispanic people typically have _____ skin that is usually characterized by more oil production.

SKIN TYPES VERSUS SKIN CONDITIONS

Short Answer

Name at least 13 of the most common skin conditions that an esthetician focuses on.

1. _____

2. _____

3. _____

4. _____

5. _____

6. _____

7. _____

8. _____

9. _____

10. _____

11. _____

12. _____

13. _____

SKIN CONDITIONS

Matching

Match the following terms with their descriptions below.

1. dehydration — redness, distended capillaries from weakening of the capillary walls

2. actinic keratosis — mass of hardened sebum and skin cells in a hair follicle; an open comedone or blackhead when exposed to oxygen. Closed comedones are whiteheads that are blocked and do not have a follicular opening.

3. telangiectasias — lack of water

4. enlarged pores — acne breakouts from hormonal changes or other factors

5. adult acne — expansions due to elasticity loss or trauma

6. couperose skin — lack of oxygen

7. sun damage — excessive buildup of dead skin cells/ keratinized cells

8. comedone — distended capillaries from weakening of the capillary walls

9. hyperkeratinization — rough area that appears from sun exposure; may have a layered scale or scab that sometimes falls off

10. pustules — discoloration from melanin production due to sun, other factors, or irritation

11. asphyxiated — infected papule with fluid inside

12. erythema — large blackheads around the eyes from sun exposure

13. cysts — lines and damage from internal or external causes

14. solar comedones — UV damage to the epidermis and dermis

15. milia — fluid, infection, or other matter under the skin

16. wrinkles/aging — hardened whiteheads with no visible opening

17. hyperpigmentation — redness caused by inflammation

18. keratosis/keratoses	white, colorless areas from lack of melanin production
19. sensitivities	raised lesions/blemishes
20. seborrhea	vascular disorder; chronic redness; papules and pustules may be present
21. papules	buildup of cells; a rough texture
22. poor elasticity	usually redness or inflammation from a variety of causes
23. irritation	reactions from internal or external causes
24. hypopigmentation	severe oiliness of the skin
25. rosacea	sagging; loose skin from damage, sun, and aging

HEALTHY HABITS FOR THE SKIN

True/False

Keeping your skin healthy is something that you should not only speak with your clients about; you should also follow your own advice. Write *true* next to the correct healthy habits and *false* next to the incorrect ones.

True/False   **1.** Avoid sun exposure.

_____

True/False   **2.** Eating hamburgers and hot dogs is healthy for your skin.

_____

True/False   **3.** Do not smoke.

_____

True/False   **4.** Avoid excessive alcohol.

_____

True/False   **5.** Drink a minimal amount of water.

_____

True/False   **6.** Get five hours of rest at night.

_____

True/False   **7.** Stay active and exercise regularly.

_____

True/False	8. Use beneficial products and home care.

_____

True/False	9. You don't need to get facials for good skin maintenance.

_____

True/False	10. Avoid stress and maintain a calm, positive attitude.

_____

CONTRAINDICATIONS

Short Essay

Describe the common contraindications and related precautions for skin treatments in the space provided below.

- _____

  _____

- _____

  _____

- _____

  _____

- _____

  _____

- _____

  _____

- _____

  _____

- _____

  _____

- _____

  _____

- _____

  _____

- _____

  _____

- _____
  _____
- _____
  _____

CLIENT CONSULTATIONS

Short Answer

On the spaces below, list some of the questions you should ask while performing a client consultation.

- _____
  _____
- _____
  _____
- _____
  _____
- _____
  _____
- _____
  _____
- _____
  _____
- _____
  _____

Can you think of any other important questions that you should ask your clients?

_____
_____
_____

PERFORMING A SKIN ANALYSIS

Short Essay

After reading the following scenarios, answer the question at the end of each paragraph.

_____

_____

1. A 25-year-old woman comes in for a facial, and she complains of shiny skin that often has breakouts. She is hoping that you can help her acne issues. What do you think you would observe under the magnifying lamp?

_____

_____

_____

_____

_____

2. A 40-year-old man comes in and is complaining of dry, flaky skin. As you look at his skin, you observe blackheads around his eyes and chin. What do you think the best procedure for him would be?

_____

_____

_____

_____

_____

3. A woman comes in for a facial and she is in her mid-30s. She has some hyperpigmentation on her upper lip and is concerned about it getting darker. What could you sell to her to help correct the problem?

_____

_____

_____

_____

_____

4. A mother comes in with her 16-year-old daughter so the daughter can receive a treatment. The daughter has pustules and blackheads around her mouth, chin, and forehead. What type of facial procedure should she receive and what products should you sell her?

_____

_____

_____

_____

_____

5. A mother brings her son in to receive some advice. The son is 17 years old, plays football, and says he washes his face with antibacterial soap. He has acne on his forehead and cheeks and around his nose yet his skin seems to be a bit dry and flaky. What type of skin does he have?

_____

_____

_____

_____

_____

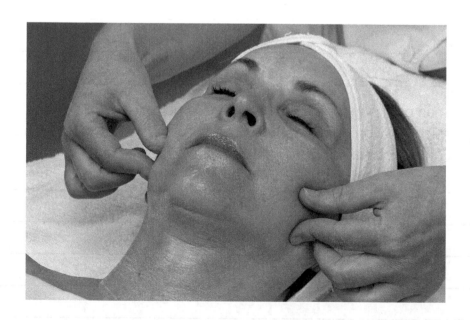

© Milady, a part of Cengage Learning.
Photography by Larry Hamill.

CHAPTER

13 Skin Care Products: Chemistry, Ingredients, and Selection

Date: _____

Rating: _____

WHY STUDY SKIN CARE PRODUCTS: CHEMISTRY, INGREDIENTS, AND SELECTION?

Short Essay

Why should estheticians have a thorough understanding of skin care products? Please provide your answer below.

_____

_____

_____

_____

_____

_____

_____

_____

_____

_____

_____

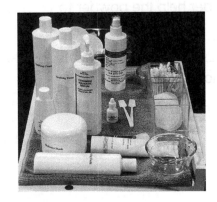

COSMETIC CHEMISTRY

Fill in the Blank

Fill in the blank with the correct answer.

1. The Food and Drug Administration (_____) views cosmetics according to the _____, which distinguishes between _____.

2. _____ are defined by the FDA as "articles that are intended to be rubbed, poured, sprinkled or otherwise applied to the human body or any part thereof for cleansing, beautifying, promoting attractiveness or alternating the appearance."

3. _____ allow products to spread, give them body and texture, and give them a specific form such as a lotion, cream, or gel.

4. _____ cause the actual changes in the appearance of skin.

5. _____ are a proposed third category; they are intended to improve the skin's health and appearance.

6. Ingredients can be derived from _____.

7. _____ describes ingredients that may be less likely to cause allergic reactions.

8. _____ describes ingredients that will not clog pores or cause comedones.

9. _____ is the most frequently used cosmetic ingredient.

10. As a performance ingredient, water _____ _____.

11. Products that do not contain any water are called _____.

12. Fatty materials used to lubricate and moisturize the face are called _____.

13. Emollients in loose powder help the powder to _____ _____.

14. As performance drugs, _____ lubricate the skin's surface and set up a guard for the barrier functions.

15. Mineral oil and petrolatum come from the _____.

16. Plant oils contain _____, which are beneficial for skin that does not produce enough sebum.

17. _____ are lubricant ingredients derived from plant oils or animal fats.

18. When fatty acids have been exposed to hydrogen, they become _____.

19. _____ are produced from fatty acids and fatty alcohols.

21. Dimethicone, cyclomethicone, and phenyl trimethicone are examples of _____.

22. Comedogenicity is the tendency of any topical substance to cause or to worsen a _____.

23. Which category of ingredients reduces the surface tension between the skin and the product? _____

24. The main type of surfactant used in cleansing agents is _____.

25. _____ is the therapeutic use of plant aromas and essential oils for beauty and health treatment purposes.

26. _____ prevent bacteria and other microorganisms from living in a product.

27. A _____ is added to products to improve the efficiency of a preservative.

28. The _____ regulates color agent ingredients.

29. Certified colors are listed on ingredient labels as _____.

30. Insoluble pigments made by combining a dye with an inorganic material are _____.

32. Exfoliation can be achieved through _____ actions.

33. _____ physically scrape dead cells from the skin's surface.

34. Alpha hydroxy acids are used to _____ exfoliate the skin.

35. Papain, bromelain, and pancreatin are all _____ that gently exfoliate the skin.

36. _____ are ingredients used in the bleaching or lightening of the skin.

37. _____ converts tyrosine into melanin.

38. _____ deliver ingredients to specific tissues of the epidermis.

39. Water and emollients are _____ that carry other ingredients into the skin.

40. What are liposomes? What is their purpose? _____

_____

_____

41. Which delivery system releases substances onto the skin's surface at a microscopically controlled rate? _____

42. What is the proper name for microsponges? _____

43. Vitamins C and E, green tea, and DMAE are _____.

44. Polyglucans are _____; they help preserve and protect collagen and elastin.

45. Beta-glucans help reduce the appearance of fine lines and wrinkles by

_____.

46. _____ is derived from yeast cells and functions as an anti-inflammatory and moisturizing ingredient.

47. Glycoproteins are derived from _____.

48. _____ are chains of amino acids used in skin care products to produce changes in the appearance of the skin.

49. _____ is a natural form of Vitamin A.

50. Retinoic acid is a form of Vitamin A that is of the keratolytic group. What does this mean? _____

51. Vitamins C and E, alphalipoic acid, idebenone, and coenzyme Q-10 are all

_____.

52. There are two types of sunscreen ingredients: _____.

53. Chemical sunscreens chemically _____ ultraviolet rays.

54. The FDA regulates cosmetics in terms of _____, _____, and

_____.

55. Cosmetic ingredients are listed in _____ order of predominance, starting with the ingredient that has the _____ concentration.

56. What should you do after applying a product if the skin becomes excessively red or the client complains of burning? _____

_____

57. Before a treatment, it is a good idea to _____ any client who has reactive skin.

58. Aromatherapy is a(n) _____ healing practice.

59. Aromatherapy treats the _____.

60. _____ is the use of plant extracts for therapeutic benefits.

61. _____ are the main focus of the skin care industry.

62. _____ neutralize the damaging effects of free radicals.

63. Vitamin C strengthens the _____ and is essential for producing _____.

64. Dimethylaminoethanol is commonly called _____.

65. Vitamins A and E protect the _____.

Matching

Match the following terms with their descriptions below.

hydrators	botanicals/phytotherapy
pH adjusters	solvents

1. _____: alkaline and acid bases that adjust the pH of products

2. _____: ingredients derived from plants that benefit the skin

3. _____: also known as humectants

4. _____: substances such as water that are used to dissolve other ingredients

PRODUCT COMPONENTS

Short Answer

Answer the following questions.

1. Explain how alpha hydroxy acids and beta hydroxy acids work.

   _____

2. How do enzymes exfoliate the skin? _____

   _____

   _____

3. List some of the common lightening agents. _____

   _____

   _____

4. What are three types of ingredient delivery systems? _____

_____

5. How do beta-glucans and polyglucans benefit the skin? _____

_____

_____

_____

6. What is a keratolytic derived from Vitamin A? _____

VITAMINS AND ANTIOXIDANTS

Short Answer

Answer the following questions.

1. How do antioxidants help the skin? _____

_____

_____

2. Describe a free radical. _____

_____

_____

3. As an antioxidant, what is the benefit of Vitamin C? _____

_____

4. What is the benefit of alpha lipoic acid? _____

_____

_____

5. What is the benefit of CoQ10? _____

_____

_____

6. What are three types of organic chemical sunscreens? _____

_____

7. What are two types of inorganic physical sunscreens? _____

_____

INGREDIENTS

Matching

Match these ingredients to their definitions.

urea	collagen	benzoyl peroxide
ceramides	squalene	salicylic acid
petroleum jelly	peptides	methylparaben
alcohol	hyaluronic acid	lanolin
propylene glycol	mineral oil	

_____

_____

_____

_____

_____

_____

_____

_____

1. occlusive agent that restores the barrier layer by holding in water; used after laser surgery to protect the skin while healing
2. antiseptic and solvent used in perfumes, lotions, and astringents
3. glycolipid materials that are a natural part of skin's intercellular matrix and barrier function
4. properties include enhancing the penetration abilities of other substances and anti-inflammatory, antiseptic, and deodorizing action that protects the skin's surface and helps maintain healthy skin
5. emollient with moisturizing properties; also an emulsifier with high water absorption capabilities
6. chains of amino acids that stimulate fibroblasts, cell metabolism, collagen, and improve skin's firmness; larger chains are called polypeptides
7. one of the most frequently used preservatives because of its very low sensitizing potential; combats bacteria and molds; noncomedogenic
8. fibrous, connective tissue made from protein; found in the reticular layer of the dermis; gives skin its firmness; topically, a large, long-chain molecular protein that lies on the top of the skin and binds water; derived from the placentas of cows or other sources

_____ **9.** lubricant derived from petroleum

_____ **10.** a humectant often used in dry or sensitive skin moisturizers

_____ **11.** originally from shark liver oil; also occurs in small amounts in olive oil, wheat germ oil, and rice bran oil; also found in human sebum; a lubricant and perfume fixative

_____ **12.** drying ingredient with antibacterial properties commonly used for blemishes and acne

_____ **13.** hydrating fluids found in the skin; hydrophilic agent with water-binding properties

_____ **14.** beta hydroxy acid with exfoliating and antiseptic properties; natural sources include sweet birch, willow bark, and wintergreen

AROMATHERAPY

True/False

Determine whether the following statements are true or false.

T F **1.** Aromatherapy is a new practice that uses essential oils and aromas from plants to only treat physical ailments.

T F **2.** Phytotherapy uses oil extracts for therapeutic benefits.

T F **3.** Our sense of smell is called the olfactory system.

T F **4.** Aromatherapy scents are massage oils.

T F **5.** An aromatherapy massage can be created by adding essential oils to massage oils, creams, and lotions.

MATURE SKIN

Short Answer

Many ingredients are available to support the needs of mature skin. List the ingredients that have proven to have a positive effect on mature skin and rosacea.

- _____

- _____

- _____

- _____

- _____

- _____
- _____
- _____
- _____
- _____

PRODUCT SELECTION

Short Answer

Answer the following questions appropriately.

1. Name the main categories in skin care products.

   a) _____

   b) _____

   c) _____

   d) _____

   e) _____

   f) _____

   g) _____

2. Cleansers should leave the skin _____ balanced.

3. Cleansers _____ makeup and dirt to keep _____ clean and _____ for other products.

4. What are the three basic forms of cleansers?

   a) _____

   b) _____

   c) _____

5. Describe the purpose of a cleansing gel. _____

   _____

6. What is the most important caution to consider when recommending a cleansing gel? _____

7. Describe a cleansing lotion. _____

   _____

8. Milky cleansing lotions are used by which skin type? _____

9. Describe the purposes of a cleansing cream. _____

_____

10. Are makeup removers generally oil-based or water-based? _____

11. _____ usually have a higher alcohol content and are designed for use on normal and combination skin.

12. _____ have the highest alcohol content and are used for oily and acne-prone skin.

13. List at least 8 general benefits of exfoliating the skin.

a) _____

b) _____

c) _____

d) _____

e) _____

f) _____

g) _____

h) _____

14. List the skin conditions that benefit from exfoliation.

a) _____

_____

b) _____

_____

c) _____

_____

15. What does exfoliation refer to? _____

_____

16. _____ is a method of physically rubbing dead cells off the skin.

17. _____ dissolves the intercellular glue by using chemical agents such as AHAs.

18. How do enzymes remove dead skin cells? _____

_____

19. Contraindications for harsh mechanical peel techniques, scrubs, and brushing machines include:

a) _____

b) _____

c) _____

d) _____

e) _____

f) _____

_____

20. Gommage is a cream type of _____ peel that is removed by

_____.

21. Masks and packs offer many benefits. List seven advantages of using these products.

a) _____

b) _____

c) _____

d) _____

e) _____

f) _____

g) _____

22. Clay masks draw _____ to the surface of the skin as they dry and

_____.

23. Alginate masks are often _____ based and dry to form a _____ texture.

24. When do you apply serums and ampoules? _____

_____

25. Why do serums penetrate deeper into the skin? _____

_____

26. What are ampoules? _____

_____

27. List the benefits of eye creams.

  a) _____

  b) _____

  c) _____

  d) _____

28. _____ include moisturizing balms and products with collagen derivatives to _____ up the lips.

29. Lotions, hydrators, and creams are known as _____

30. Oil-based moisturizers contain _____ They are heavier and occlusive to _____ and _____ under the cream.

31. Why does oily skin need hydration? _____

_____

_____

32. Treatment creams and massage lotions are different forms of _____.

33. Treatment creams are often _____ in consistency than moisturizers and contain more _____ and _____ ingredients.

34. What six negative results can occur when the skin is not protected from ultraviolet rays?

  a) _____

  b) _____

  c) _____

  d) _____

  e) _____

  f) _____

35. Sunscreens _____ UV rays.

HOME CARE PRODUCTS

Short Essay

Answer the following questions. Then conduct a short survey to practice your sales skills.

1. What was your home care regimen before you started school?

_____

_____

_____

_____

_____

2. What do you currently use for your cleanser, toner, and moisturizer?

_____

_____

_____

_____

_____

3. Survey three people and write down what they currently use for home-care products; then make recommendations for what they should be using.

Survey 1: _____

_____

_____

Survey 2: _____

_____

_____

Survey 3: _____

_____

_____

SKIN CARE PRODUCTS

Word Search

Find the words in the word bank within the word search below.

astringents	emollients	olfactory
allantoin	fresheners	papaya
binders	glycerin	polyglucans
calendula	green tea	squalane
ceramides	jojoba	sulfur
cosmetics	lakes	urea

```
W L G T H P F L Q P H A G A Y A P A P D
V A L L A N T O I N V Q O B L U Q S A T
T D N C L U G D N K A S D P A T C C B Z
J T G R E E N T E A S B O U Q G A I I N
F S F D Q O V P G U N P C K P E W T N Q
A T G O V F O S E D I M A R E C E E D Y
U N A J P Q N L W U Y B U S F Q N M E F
Q E R N F V A C B Y T O N W N Q J S R S
T I J L P C I D R S F A M A Q K E O S R
J L P O F T Z O A N C J B E P E A C B E
T L C V B M T R F U G E N B S D B S P N
C O P Q F C D J L H V A T E E M O B N E
U M T U A C Q G T D L U K Y Z D J D R H
Q E J F I S Y U P A T A A T J U O F U S
F J L T F L B Z U S L S F R D T J U H E
G O F R O C R Q R P D H U P Q N Z S P R
U F Z P Q J S N F A L U D N E L A C L F
R I D T U I W O E E Z O M B S M R D U Q
E R N I R E C Y L G O P D P G D M B S M
A F L D N F D A S T R I N G E N T S D Q
```

© Milady, a part of Cengage Learning.

CHAPTER **14** **The Treatment Room**

Date: _____

Rating: _____

WHY STUDY THE TREATMENT ROOM?

Short Essay

On the lines below, explain why an esthetician should have a thorough understanding of the treatment room.

_____

_____

_____

_____

_____

_____

_____

_____

_____

_____

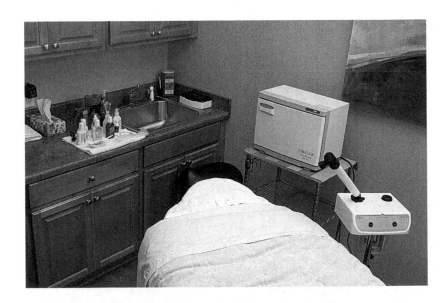

THE ESTHETICIAN'S PRESENTATION AND FURNITURE, EQUIPMENT, AND ROOM SETUP

Fill in the Blank

Place the appropriate word or phrase on the lines provided.

1. Why is making a good first impression important? _____

_____

2. Being dependable and providing excellent customer service is _____ .

3. Creating a _____, comfortable, and relaxing atmosphere is part of your service.

4. What is another name for a treatment table? _____

5. The esthetician's stool should be _____ correct.

6. A hot towel cabinet is mainly used to heat up towels but could also be used for

_____ .

7. What is the magnifying lamp used for? _____

8. What is the purpose of a steamer? _____

9. A wet disinfectant should be located in each treatment room for disinfecting tools and equipment. Implements must be thoroughly _____ of all visible matter _____ being placed in disinfectant solution.

10. What is the wax heater used for? _____

_____

11. A laundry container should be _____ .

12. What is another name for a sharp's container? _____

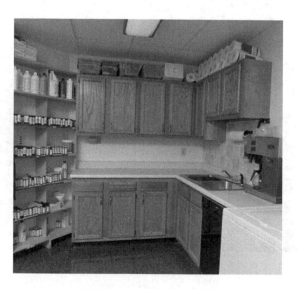

FACIAL SUPPLIES

Mind Mapping

List the supplies that are needed for a facial. One has been filled in for you already.

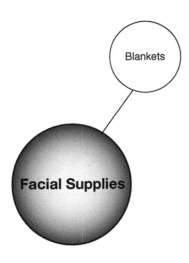

SINGLE USE ITEMS

Fill in the Blank

Single-use items are disposable and can only be used once. Using the lines provided, list five examples of single-use items below.

_____

_____

_____

_____

_____

_____

PRODUCTS

Word Search

Find the products needed for a facial in the word search.

cleanser	sunscreens	serums
face massage	lip balm	mask
cream	exfoliant	moisturizer
lotion	toner	eye cream
	astringent	

```
Q C L E A N S E R N H A N O I T O L O B
X C P K C K Z X V J O Q O B L U Q T M U
U S U N S C R E E N S T D P C T C A H G
G T I T G Q O H N B T B O U T G S J C V
O T G E R O V N M U N P C K P K W N H Q
T U F N W F O V B E J N R S J C E V L Y
I C R E A M N V Q U Y E U Q F Q N I F B
O A S O G V R M V Y Z O A W N E J J C X
N E L B V E I F E I F B M A G K E S X Q
K R Q K N T Z V R N D J B A P E B A N I
E C D O U M U U V T G E S B S M Q S P S
Y E T R J D T K B H V S T T L N F T V E
E Y U M V S Q J B D A U A A Z D T R B R
C E K N I T V B P M T L B T J U O I U U
R K T O B N B B E S P P F R D T N N B M
E U M R Q D S C R Q I H U P Q N E G X S
A K Z A K K A V F L G L E B O D R E S L
M T D T V F F O E E Z O M B S M I N O C
E S Q I S G B X V B K Q L P G D L T Y Z
Y E X F O L I A N T S G L X K T V D I B
```

PREPARING THE EQUIPMENT AND ROOM

Fill in the Blank

Put the following steps in order by placing the proper number in front of the direction.

_____ Turn on the wax heater as needed. Check and adjust the temperature.

_____ Lay out one hand towel to place under the head and one for placement over the décolleté (day-call-TAY) on the upper chest area if applicable.

_____ Place clean linens neatly on the treatment table.

_____ Place a blanket on top of the linens to keep the client warm and comfortable.

_____ Preheat the towel warmer and put in wet towels.

_____ Preheat the steamer.

_____ Have a bolster and pillow available.

_____ Wash your hands with soap and warm water before setting up and touching clean items.

_____ Preheat any other equipment needed.

_____ Have a clean headband and gown or wrap ready for the client.

_____ Check to make sure the disinfectant is ready. Wet disinfectants are filled and changed according to manufacturer's instructions (check to see that the strength is maintained by regular refilling).

_____ Place supplies on a clean towel (paper or cloth) on the clean and disinfected workstation. (Put out supplies in the order used, lined up neatly, and cover with another towel until you are ready to use them.)

CLEANING AND DISINFECTING IMPLEMENTS

Fill in the Blank

The following is a list of steps for cleaning and disinfecting procedures. Fill in the missing words.

1. Wear gloves for all _____ to prevent contamination and protect hands from the strong chemicals. Wash hands after completing decontamination procedures.

2. Wash and disinfect all _____
_____ · Wash implements thoroughly with _____ and dry them off first before placing in the disinfectant. This process is important to maintain the wet disinfectant strength and keep it from becoming dirty or diluted.

3. Be sure all implements remain in the disinfectant for the _____
_____ . Remove with tongs;
then _____ , dry, and put them away.

4. Store clean items in a _____ in a drawer or cupboard when not
in use.

5. Clean and disinfect bowls and other multi-use items. _____ properly.

6. Change the _____ to comply with manufacturer's directions and
regulations. If required, record on a dated log when the disinfectant is
changed.

END OF DAY CLEAN-UP

Fill in the Blank

Following is a checklist for the end of the day. Fill in the missing steps in the spaces
provided.

☐ Use a clean-up checklist to make sure you did not forget anything.

☐ _____

☐ Leave the towel-warmer door open to dry, and empty the tray underneath before
cleaning and disinfecting it.

☐ _____

_____

☐ Refill all containers, supplies, and the steamer.

☐ _____

☐ _____

☐ Remove personal items from the area.

SAVING MONEY AND RESOURCES WITH GREEN PRACTICES

Short Essay

Write an essay in which you discuss the various ways you can make your salon
more cost efficient and create a more "green" environment.

_____

_____

_____

_____

_____

_____

_____

_____

_____

_____

_____

_____

_____

RESOURCES

Word Scramble

Unscramble the word to match the definition.

1. mmitspleen   Tools used by technicians. _____

2. ytissulnaitab   Meeting the needs of the present without compromising the ability of future generations to meet their needs. The three facets of sustainability are the three Es: the Environment, the Economy, and social Equity. _____

3. psrahs ctrnoneai   Plastic biohazard container for disposable needles and anything sharp. The container is red and puncture-proof and must be disposed of as medical waste. _____

4. SHOAL   Acronym for Lifestyle of Health and Sustainability; forward-thinking consumers who consider the impact on the environment and society when making purchasing decisions. _____

5. ysdirpaien   Room or area used for mixing products and storing supplies. _____

15 Facial Treatments

Date: _____

Rating: _____

WHY STUDY FACIAL TREATMENTS?

Short Essay

Needless to say, facial treatments make up a very large portion of our profession. What do you think the most important parts of the facial treatment studies are? Provide your answer on the lines below.

_____

_____

_____

_____

_____

FACIAL TREATMENT BENEFITS

Short Answer

List the benefits of a facial treatment.

- _____

- _____

- _____

- _____

- _____

- _____

- _____

- _____

- _____

SKIN HISTOLOGY

Mind Mapping

Using the mind map, write the skills that are needed to be successful at giving facials.

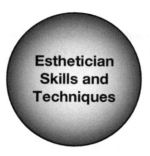

Esthetician
Skills and
Techniques

KEY ELEMENTS OF THE BASIC FACIAL TREATMENT

Fill in the Blank

Write down the steps into which a basic facial is divided. Some have been provided for you.

1. _____

2. _____

3. _____

4. In-depth skin analysis (refer to Table 15-3 in your textbook)

5. _____

6. _____

7. _____

8. Massage

9. _____

10. _____

11. _____

Now create a list for the contraindications of a facial. Some answers have been provided for you.

12. _____

13. _____

14. _____

15. _____

16. Use of acne drugs or other topical peeling agents

17. Skin irritation

18. _____

19. _____

20. _____

TOWEL DRAPING

Label the Image

In the space provided, describe the steps involved in towel draping in the photos.

_____

_____

_____

_____

_____

_____

_____

_____

_____

_____

_____

FACIAL TREATMENTS

Fill in the Blank

State the appropriate answer in the lines provided for each of the following statements or questions.

1. Products that should be used for lip color removal are _____.

2. When removing lip products, begin with the _____

   _____.

3. What three benefits are found in the exfoliation process?

   a) _____

   b) _____

   c) _____

4. Heat applied through steam or warm towels accomplishes what five things?

   a) _____

   b) _____

   c) _____

   d) _____

   e) _____

5. Name the three methods for doing extractions.

   a) _____

   b) _____

   c) _____

6. You must always wear _____ when doing extractions.

7. _____ are metal tools used for open comedones and sebaceous filaments.

8. The skin must be _____ and _____ before extractions.

9. If extractions are done improperly, the follicle walls can rupture and

   _____.

10. Proper cleansing is essential when extracting blemishes to avoid

    _____.

11. Once the skin becomes dry and resistive, _____ doing extractions.

12. List the areas of the face where the follicles are perpendicular to the surface of the skin.

a) _____

b) _____

c) _____

d) _____

13. Other areas of the skin, such as the nose and cheeks, have _____.

14. A small, sharp, pointed surgical blade with a double edge is called a _____.

15. Most clients will tolerate approximately _____ minutes of extraction.

16. Describe the proper use of a lancet when opening closed comedones.

_____

_____

17. Describe the benefits of a treatment mask.

a) _____

b) _____

c) _____

d) _____

e) _____

f) _____

18. Depending on their function, masks are applied _____

_____.

19. Toners hydrate and finish the cleansing process by _____

_____.

20. _____ are concentrated liquid ingredients used for specific corrective treatments.

21. Depending on the skin condition, moisturizers can:

a) _____

b) _____

c) _____

22. After finishing a stimulating, nourishing facial, do not send your client out without _____.

23. Antibacterial products and the high-frequency machine kill _____ and help _____.

24. After completing the facial service, quietly and slowly let the client know you are _____.

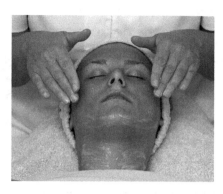

BASIC FACIAL TREATMENT

Fill in the Blank

Match the following terms with their descriptions below.

contraindications	steps	infection control
draping	rejuvenate	serums
extractions	remove	time
facial sponges	mini-facial	

1. A facial is a professional service designed to improve and _____ the skin.

2. _____ are conditions that prevent a client from receiving a treatment.

3. _____ the client refers to adjusting the head drape, towels, and linens.

4. Because foam and gel cleansers are harder to _____, it is advisable to use a milky or creamy cleanser that rinses easily during a facial.

5. While cleansing, some estheticians prefer to use wet cotton pads and others choose to use _____.

6. The skin must be exfoliated and warmed before _____.

7. _____ are concentrated ingredients used for specific treatments.

8. Performing your _____ procedures in your clients' presence will make them feel more confident in you as a professional.

9. The main differences between a _____ and a basic facial are the _____ and number of _____.

TREATMENTS FOR DIFFERENT SKIN TYPES AND CONDITIONS

Fill in the Blank

Fill in the blanks with the appropriate words. Some sentences may have more than one answer.

1. Dry skin can appear to be _____ but feel _____ to the touch.

2. Treatment goals are similar for dry and _____ skin.

3. When treating dry skin, use a(n) _____ _____ to exfoliate the face.

4. When treating dry skin, _____ masks can be used.

5. Moisturizing creams with a(n) _____ base are recommended for dry skin types.

6. Skin may have a sufficient amount of oil but still feel dry and flaky due to _____.

7. When treating dehydrated skin, employ treatments that are similar to the ones for _____ skin.

8. Extreme weight loss can result in loss of _____ and _____.

9. Exposure to extreme climates and too much sun, wind, or polluted air will _____.

10. Mature clients' skin can be improved, but the natural aging process cannot be _____.

11. Treatment goals for mature skin are to _____.

12. When treating mature skin, a(n) _____ will plump and force-feed nutrients into the skin.

13. The primary goal when treating sensitive skin is to _____ the skin.

14. Aloe vera, chamomile, allantoin, azulene, and licorice extracts are all effective on _____ skin.

15. Individuals with sensitive skin should avoid stimulating, drying products and _____.

16. Rosacea, like seborrhea, can be characterized by _____ of the skin.

17. A gentle cleanser, less steam and heat, an enzyme peel, and a soothing gel mask are recommended products/procedures for _____.

18. The best preventive measure for hyperpigmentation is _____ _____.

19. Brighteners such as kojic acid, mulberry, licorice root, bearberry, and azaleic acid are known to _____.

20. Oily and combination skins need _____ products.

21. Acne facials concentrate on clearing the follicles by _____ _____.

22. Oxygen masks, glycolic acid peels, sulfur masks, anti-inflammatory masks, steaming, extractions, and desincrustation are all treatments recommended for _____.

23. Benzoyl peroxide releases free radical oxygen that kills _____ and sterilizes the _____.

24. Before recommending a salicylic mask, the esthetician must check for _____ allergies.

25. Cleaning out the debris that expands them allows the pores to _____.

SKIN TYPE

Fill in the Blank

Use the terms provided to match the following terms with their descriptions below.

occlusive	oil	serum
body	metabolism	physiological
antioxidant	hydration	oil-based
dry	natural	paraffin

1. _____ products are necessary to protect and balance dry skin.

2. Skin is often lacking _____ due to inactivity of the sebaceous glands.

3. The purpose of treatments for dry or mature skin is to stimulate the cell _____.

4. Dry skin requires a(n) _____ cream.

5. _____ skin benefits from collagen, hydrating, paraffin wax, or thermal masks.

6. Dry skin is often due to the _____ aging process.

7. _____ disease, poor health, and psychological problems can cause the skin to appear older.

8. Sodium hyaluronate and sodium PCA enhance _____.

9. Vitamins C and E as well as grapeseed extract have _____ properties.

10. The _____ mask can be applied in a facial or alone.

11. A(n) _____ is used under the mask for specific skin conditions.

12. Melt the paraffin in a warming unit to a little more than _____ temperature.

SKIN TREATMENTS

True/False

Determine whether each statement is true or false and explain your answer in the space provided.

T   F   **1.** Hydroquinone is one of many FDA-approved hyperpigmentation treatments.

_____

_____

_____

T   F   **2.** Brighteners such as kojic acid, mulberry, and bearberry are known to reduce pigmentation.

_____

_____

_____

T   F   **3.** In treatments, the suction and the brush machine are too irritating for sensitive skin.

_____

_____

_____

T   F   **4.** Acne treatments may include alpha hydroxy acids, beta hydroxy acids, and sulfur masks.

_____

_____

_____

_____

T   F   **5.** Oil-free products are noncomedogenic.

_____

_____

_____

ACNE TREATMENT CARE

Word Search

Answer the following questions to obtain the correct word for the word search puzzle.

_____   What is a beta hydroxy acid that is helpful for acne?

_____   What is a type of mask that is good for acne that will help exfoliate skin and heal and dry blemishes?

_____   This oral vitamin has antioxidant value and healing effects.

_____   This vitamin that starts with the letter z is also helpful in fighting acne.

_____   Glycolic and tartaric are examples of this type of acid.

_____   This product releases free radical oxygen that kills the bacteria that causes acne.

_____   This type of product reduces bacteriaand can also oxygenate and open impacted follicles for easier extractions.

_____   These types of products can clog pores.

_____   What other environmental aggravators besides dirt, grease, sun, and humidity can affect the skin?

_____   What are individual finger gloves called?

```
V C M V I B Y Y P A R E H T N E G Y X O
C A H A S K Z X B J N M K M L U M T N C
N P K D J F I N G E R C O T S T C C H V
M T I T G Q O H N X T B O U T G B J E V
V T G E R O V N V U N P C K P M W D H Q
C U D N W F O V B E J N J K J C I G L P
N C I K Q R N V Q U Y C S Q F X N K G O
L J C O G V A M V Y Z A A W O Q J N M L
J S A B V C I F E V M B M R X K C P X L
V N C K V T Z V J R D J E P P O B C N U
X D I T U M U X U T G P F B M D Q S P T
N J L R J D C F B H L X T E E N F B V I
V K Y M V W L J B Y J U D Y Z D C D B O
I F C N M U V B O S T O A T J C B F U N
G X I X S N B Z U S G S F R D T M U Z X
B J L R Q D N X R E D H U P Q N Z Z I H
S S A A K E V N N B G L E B X D Z V N X
V U S T B J F I E E Z O M B S M J X C X
C J Q I S G C X V B K Q L P G D F A Y A
Y C J L C N K C N I M A T I V B C E J C
```

MEN'S SKIN CARE

Fill in the Blank

Fill in the blank spaces for the following statements with the correct words or phrases.

1. List the key points to consider when choosing skin care products for men.

   a) _____

   b) _____

2. What type of protective clothing do men wear during a treatment? _____

   _____

3. Men want a _____ routine.

4. Using the term _____ rather than facial is a better way to promote men's services.

5. Men typically have larger _____ and _____ than women do.

6. Men prefer simple routines and _____ products.

7. When working with men, tubes and pumps are more male-friendly than _____.

8. Cotton pads or gauze will _____. _____ are more appropriate for a man's face.

9. _____ is often referred to as razor bumps.

10. Pseudofolliculitis resembles folliculitis without the _____.

MEN'S FACIAL

True/False

Determine whether the following statements are true or false and explain your answer in the space provided.

T   F   1. Professional movements during a man's facial should flow against the hair growth.

_____

_____

T   F   2. Men need brisk products so they can feel the results of your services.

_____

_____

T   F   3. Pseudofolliculitis is characterized by bumps that are filled with pus.

_____

_____

T   F   4. A man's home-care regimen should initially include only two products.

_____

_____

PARAFFIN MASK PROCEDURE

Fill in the Blank

Fill in the blanks with the correct numbers. Put the steps in the correct order by placing the correct number next to the procedure.

_____ 1. Test the temperature of the paraffin by applying to the inside of the wrist with a spatula. Discard any used wax in a plastic bag for waste disposal.

_____ 2. After draping and cleansing, place eye pads on client.

_____ 3. Continue adding layers of paraffin to the top of the gauze until the application is approximately ¼-inch (0.6 centimeters) thick. The application of wax will take approximately 10 minutes.

_____ 4. Melt the paraffin in a warming unit to a little more than body temperature (98.6 degrees Fahrenheit or 37 degrees Celsius). The wax may take up to an hour to heat to the proper temperature.

_____ 5. Cut the gauze to the desired size, and place it over the face and neck. It is not usually necessary to cut holes for the eyes and nose because the gauze is woven very loosely. Occasionally, however, a client may feel claustrophobic. In that case, make slits in the gauze for the eyes, nose, and mouth before use. Precut gauze pads are available and are more efficient for this use.

_____ 6. Carefully lift the mask from the neck in one piece.

_____ 7. Apply the first coat of paraffin over the gauze with a brush, beginning at the base of the neck and working up to the forehead. Do not get wax in the hair as it is difficult to get out. Use a new spatula or brush for each layer to avoid contamination by double-dipping.

_____ 8. Apply an appropriate product, such as a serum or hydrating mask, under the paraffin mask.

_____ 9. After the wax application is completed, have the client relax until the wax is hardened and ready to remove (approximately 15 minutes).

_____ 10. Finish the service with the appropriate products (toner, moisturizer).

_____ 11. When ready to remove the mask, use a wooden spatula to work the edges of the mask loose from the face and neck.

CHAPTER 16 Facial Massage

Date: ____________________

Rating: ____________________

WHY STUDY FACIAL MASSAGE?

Short Essay

Why is it important for estheticians to have a thorough understanding of facial massage? Provide answers below.

____

____

____

____

____

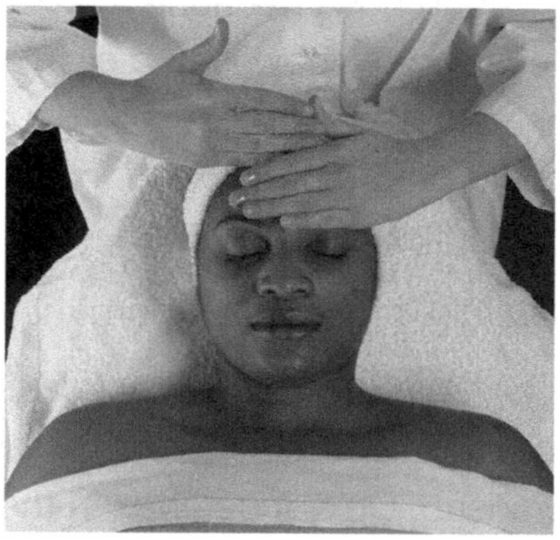

© Milady, a part of Cengage Learning. Photography by Paul Castle, Castle Photography.

THE BENEFITS OF MASSAGE

Short Answer

List the benefits that a massage gives. Some have been provided for you.

- It relaxes the client and the facial muscles.
- ______________________________________
- ______________________________________
- ______________________________________

- _____
- _____
- _____
- It helps product absorption.

- _____
- _____

INCORPORATING MASSAGE DURING THE FACIAL TREATMENT

Fill in the Blank

Place the appropriate answer in the lines provided.

1. A facial massage is performed for approximately _____ minutes during a facial.

2. Massage techniques also depend on the client's _____ and what you are focusing on in the treatment.

3. _____ is important when giving a massage.

4. _____ is important in maintaining a smooth rhythm and regulating the massage pressure.

5. What are five conditions of the body or skin that would contraindicate massage?

   a) _____

   b) _____

   c) _____

   d) _____

   e) _____

6. List five massage movements used in massage.

   a) _____

   b) _____

   c) _____

   d) _____

   e) _____

7. The most important movement is _____ .

8. Chucking, rolling, and wringing are variations of which movement? _____

9. Generally, massage movements are directed from _____ toward the _____ of the muscle.

10. If it is necessary to remove your hands from the client's face during a massage, you should _____ .

TYPES OF MASSAGE MOVEMENTS

Matching

Draw a line to match the correct word to the definition.

friction

1. light, continuous stroking movement applied with the fingers or palms in a slow and rhythmic manner

vibration

2. kneading movement that stimulates the underlying tissues

effleurage

3. deep rubbing movement requiring pressure on the skin with the fingers or palm while moving them under an underlying structure

pertrissage

4. fast tapping, slapping, and hacking movements

tapotement or percussion

5. a rapid shaking movement using your body and shoulders to create the movement

TYPES OF MASSAGE

Fill in the Blank

Answer the following questions using the appropriate word(s) or phrase(s).

1. Three variations of friction movements are _____ .

2. Where do you use chucking, rolling, and wringing movements? _____

_____

3. _____ effleurage is used on smaller surfaces such as the _____ or _____ .

4. _____ is a form of acupressure.

5. Friction movement _____ circulation and glandular activity.

6. What movement usually begins and ends a massage sequence? _____

7. _____ is the most stimulating of the general movements and should be used carefully with discretion.

8. Describe how slapping movements are performed. _____

_____

_____

9. What part of the hands do you use when executing hacking movements?_____

_____

_____

10. The parts of the body that you use in hacking and slapping movements are the _____, _____, and _____.

11. Vibration is a highly stimulating movement and should never be used for more than a _____ in one spot.

MASSAGE TYPES

Fill in the Blank

Using the word bank, place the correct answer in the lines provided.

aromatherapy	chucking	effleurage
lymph drainage massage	rolling	vibration
friction	Dr. Jacquet movement	acupressure
wringing	petrissage	reflexology

1. _____ encourages the removal of waste from the body.

2. A kneading movement that stimulates the underlying tissues is _____.

3. As the hands are working downward, the flesh is twisted against the bones in opposite directions during _____.

4. A technique named after a European dermatologist is the _____

_____.

5. A method of applying pressure to points on the body to release muscle tension is _____.

6. Both hands moving at the same time opposite to each other, twisting the flesh up and down the bone, is referred to as _____.

7. _____ is defined as maintaining pressure on the skin while moving the fingers or palms over the underlying structures.

8. _____ is the soft, continuous stroking movement applied with the fingers and palms.

9. When the flesh is grasped in one hand and moved up and down along the bone while the other hand steadies the arm, this technique is called _____.

10. _____ is a technique that is accomplished by rapid muscular contractions in the arms.

11. _____ uses essential oils that penetrate the skin during massage movements.

12. _____ is a practice based on the belief that working on areas or reflex points found on the hands, feet, ears, and face can reduce tension in the body's corresponding organs and gland structure.

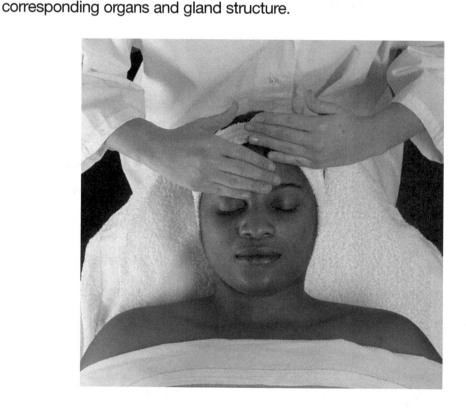

© Milady, a part of Cengage Learning. Photography by Paul Castle, Castle Photography.

SHARPENING YOUR PROFESSIONALISM

Mind Mapping

Create a "mind map" to connect the reasons a client may be unhappy to the main topic.

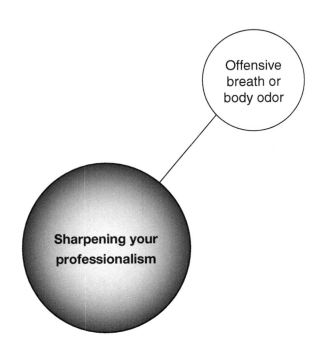

DESIGN YOUR OWN FACIAL MASSAGE

Short Essay

While including petrissage, effleurage, tapotement, vibration, and friction, create your own massage by either drawing it out step by step or write it down in your own words.

17 Facial Machines

Date: _____

Rating: _____

WHY STUDY FACIAL MACHINES?

Short Essay

Why should estheticians study and have a thorough understanding of facial machines? Provide your answer below.

_____

_____

_____

_____

_____

_____

_____

_____

_____

_____

_____

_____

_____

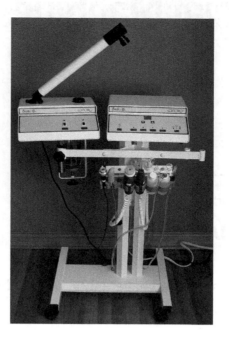

ELECTROTHERAPY

Short Answer

In the space provided, write the correct answer for each of the following.

ELECTROTHERAPY

1. Describe electrotherapy. _____

_____

2. What type of clients should electrotherapy never be used on? _____

_____

_____

_____

3. What should clients remove prior to receiving any electrotherapy?_____

_____

4. UV lamps in towel warmers may reduce bacteria, but what are they not effective for? _____

MAGNIFYING LAMP

5. What amount of magnification do magnifying lamps come in? _____

_____

6. When using the magnifying lamp, what should you loosen to position the magnifying glass so you can better analyze your client? _____

7. Why should you use eye pads when using the magnifying lamp? _____

_____

WOOD'S LAMP

8. How is the Wood's lamp different from the magnifying lamp? _____

_____

_____

9. What does the Wood's lamp show by illumination? _____

_____

WOOD'S LAMP

Matching

Draw a line connecting each color to what it means when it appears under the Wood's lamp.

1. White fluorescence	hypopigmentation
2. White spots	hyperpigmentation or sun damage
3. Blue-white	oily areas of the face/comedones
4. Light violet/purple	acne or bacteria
5. Yellow or orange	thin or dehydrated skin
6. Yellow or sometimes pink or orange	normal, healthy skin
7. Brown	horny layer of dead skin cells
8. Blue-white or yellow-green	thick corneum layer

FACIAL MACHINES

Short Answer

Answer the following questions in the spaces provided.

ROTARY BRUSH

1. What is the rotary brush used for? _____

2. If the bristles on a rotary brush become bent, what will happen?

_____

STEAMER

3. What type of water should be used in a steamer? _____

4. How far should the steamer be placed away from the client's face?

_____

5. When cleaning the steamer, how much vinegar should be added?

_____

VACUUM MACHINE

6. What are the two functions of the vacuum machine? _____

_____

7. When is it common to use the vacuum machine during a facial treatment?

_____

GALVANIC

8. Explain what the galvanic machine is for. _____

_____

9. Describe desincrustation. _____

_____

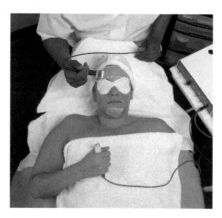

© Milady, a part of Cengage Learning. Photography by Paul Castle, Castle Photography.

10. Describe saponification. _____

_____

11. List the contraindications for galvanic current.

- _____

- _____

- _____

- _____

- _____
- _____
- _____
- _____
- _____
- _____
- _____

12. What is the difference between cataphoresis and anaphoresis?

_____

_____

HIGH FREQUENCY

13. How does high-frequency current work?

_____

_____

14. At what point during the facial treatment should high frequency be used?

_____

15. What are the benefits of high frequency?

- _____
- _____
- _____
- _____
- _____
- _____

16. What is a good rule to follow for disinfecting electrodes?

_____

_____

SPRAY MACHINE

17. What solution should be put into the machine that is partnered with the vacuum?

_____

_____

18. What type of skin should a Dr. Lucas sprayer be used on?

_____

PARAFFIN MACHINES

19. What type of skin is the paraffin treatment used for? _____

20. What is the purposed of electric mitts and boots?

_____

_____

FACIAL MACHINES

Label the Image

Name the device used on the line provided below.

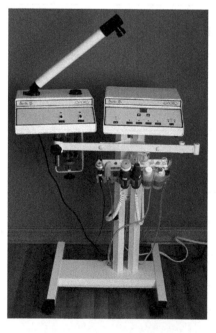

© Milady, a part of Cengage Learning. Photography by Rob Werfel.

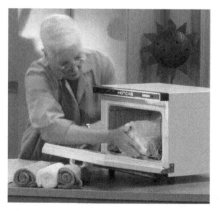

© Milady, a part of Cengage Learning. Photography by Larry Hamill.

_____   _____

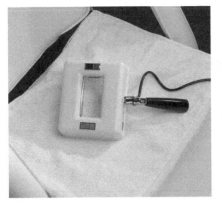

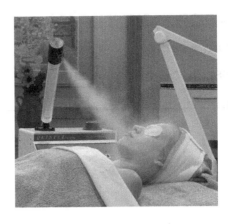

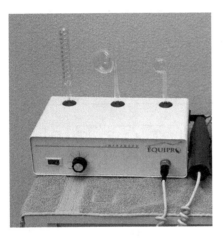

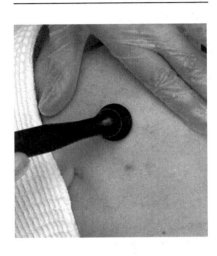

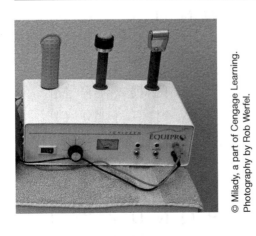

IMPORTANT TERMS
Word Search

Unscramble the terms and then locate them in the word search.

1. racaphsoeits   _____

2. eisaanhorps   _____

3. aoinnisfpoicat   _____

4. saiisuondl   _____

5. terosimlyhs   _____

6. umvauc   _____

7. spayr amnhcie   _____

8. iosinstcrudeatn   _____

9. iatonzoini   _____

10. ghhi rqucnefey iacmnhe   _____

Q	C	A	T	A	P	H	O	R	E	S	I	S	O	I	T	O	L	O	B
X	C	P	K	C	K	Z	X	V	J	O	Q	O	B	L	U	Q	T	S	U
U	A	N	A	P	H	O	R	E	S	I	S	D	P	C	N	C	I	H	G
G	T	I	T	G	Q	O	H	N	B	T	B	O	U	O	G	N	J	C	V
D	T	G	E	R	O	V	N	M	C	N	P	C	I	P	U	W	U	H	Q
E	U	F	N	W	F	O	V	I	E	J	N	T	S	S	C	E	I	L	Y
S	M	B	K	Q	R	N	F	Q	U	Y	A	U	O	F	Q	G	K	F	T
I	A	S	O	G	V	I	M	V	Y	C	O	I	W	N	H	J	S	C	H
N	E	L	B	V	N	I	F	E	I	F	D	M	A	F	K	E	S	X	E
C	R	Q	K	O	T	Z	V	F	N	A	J	B	R	P	E	P	C	N	R
R	C	D	P	U	M	U	I	V	L	G	E	E	B	S	R	Q	S	P	M
U	E	A	R	J	D	N	K	B	H	V	Q	T	T	A	N	F	B	V	O
S	S	U	M	V	O	Q	J	E	D	U	U	A	Y	Z	D	V	D	B	L
T	E	K	N	P	T	V	R	P	E	T	L	M	T	J	U	A	F	U	Y
A	K	T	A	B	N	F	B	N	S	P	A	F	R	D	T	C	U	B	S
T	U	S	R	Q	H	S	C	R	Q	C	H	U	P	Q	N	U	Z	X	I
I	K	Z	A	G	K	Y	V	F	H	G	L	E	B	O	D	U	V	K	S
O	T	D	I	V	J	F	O	I	E	Z	O	M	B	S	M	M	X	O	C
N	S	H	I	S	G	B	N	V	B	K	Q	L	P	G	D	L	N	Y	Z
Y	E	X	F	O	L	E	A	N	N	O	I	T	A	Z	I	N	O	I	B

CHAPTER 18 Hair Removal

Date: _____

Rating: _____

WHY STUDY HAIR REMOVAL?

Short Essay

On the lines below, explain what type of knowledge would an esthetician need to have to perform hair removal services?

_____

_____

_____

_____

_____

_____

_____

_____

_____

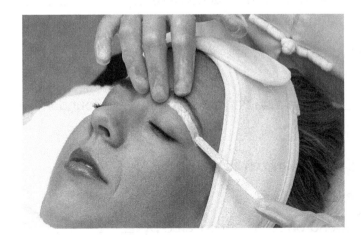

MORPHOLOGY OF THE HAIR

Short Answer

Answer the following questions in the spaces provided.

1. _____ is the study of the hair and its diseases.

2. List the main structures of the hair below the surface:

   a) _____

   b) _____

   c) _____

   d) _____

   e) _____

3. Hair is made from a hard protein called _____.

4. A pilosebaceous follicle is a mass of _____, extending down into the _____, forming a _____.

5. What is the medical term for a hair follicle? _____

6. _____ are slanted, sometimes growing in many different directions in one area.

7. The _____ are attached to the follicle.

8. The lower part of the bulb fits over and covers the _____.

9. Name the areas of the body where no hair grows. _____

   _____

10. The papilla is filled with tissue that contains _____ necessary for hair growth and nourishment of the _____.

11. When the arrector pili contracts, it makes the hair _____, causing _____.

12. _____ is the result of activity of the cells found in the basal layer.

13. Hair formation begins _____.

14. The hair on a fetus is known as _____.

15. Very soft, fine hair is called _____.

16. Vellus hair is found on areas not covered by _____ on the _____.

17. Hair grows an average of _____ per month.

18. What are the three stages of hair growth? _____

19. Which stage produces the most long-term results in terms of hair reduction?

_____

20. Hair and skin are the barometers for an individual's _____.

21. Excessive hair growth on the female body suggests a(n) _____

_____.

22. What accounts for how much hair you will normally have on your body?

_____

23. What is hirsutism? _____

_____

24. What is hypertrichosis? _____

_____

25. Hair grows faster in a _____ climate.

26. Disease, drug use, and the aging process affect the hair's _____

_____.

27. What hair growth abnormality is often associated with menopause?

_____

28. Hair protects the body from _____.

29. Individuals with olive and darker skin tones can have _____ problems
if epilation is not performed carefully.

30. Gray hair is _____ and has a deep _____.

HAIR GROWTH CYCLE

Short Answer

Answer the following questions in the spaces provided.

1. Describe the difference between the anagen, catagen, and telogen.

_____

_____

_____

2. What type of hair is found on people in the northern regions?

_____

3. What type of hair is on people from the Middle East or Mediterranean regions?

_____

4. What is the difference between hirsutism and hypertrichosis?

_____

_____

_____

5. A hormonal imbalance may also attribute to which disorder?

_____

METHODS OF HAIR REMOVAL

Matching

Match the types of hair removal with the corresponding description.

depilation

epilation

electrocoagulation

threading

electrolysis

waxing

photoepilation

sugaring

1. The only permanent method of hair removal.

2. Thermolysis is a type of this category of hair removal.

3. This method uses an intense pulsed light laser to destroy the growth cells in the hair bulb.

4. This is a process of removing hair at or near the level of the skin.

5. This is the process of removing hair from the bottom of the follicle by breaking contact between the bulb and the papilla.

6. This method works by using cotton thread that is twisted and rolled along the surface of the skin, entwining the hair in the thread and lifting it out of the follicle.

7. This is an alternative for those who have sensitive skin or who react to waxes with bumps and redness.

8. This is the primary hair removal method used by estheticians.

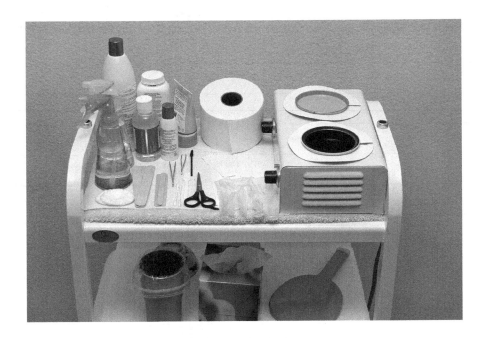

WAXING TECHNIQUES AND PRODUCTS

Short Answer

1. What are the two types of wax? _____

2. Which of those two waxes can be removed in a different direction than opposite of hair growth? _____

3. What type of wax can be used for sensitive skin? _____

4. When using soft wax, how is the wax removed? _____

5. What are some of the basic tools and supplies that should be on your cart prior to starting a service? _____

    _____

    _____

6. List the two basic contraindications for waxing.

    • _____

    _____

    • _____

    _____

7. List the six contraindications for recent treatments that a client may have had.

- _____
- _____
- _____
- _____
- _____
- _____

8. List the seven medical conditions that someone may have that would make them contraindicated to waxing.

- _____
- _____
- _____
- _____
- _____
- _____
- _____

CONTRAINDICATIONS

Mind Mapping

Using the mind map, write contraindications around the main topic.

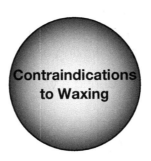

Contraindications
to Waxing

CLIENT CONSULTATIONS

Short Answer

Answer the following questions in the spaces provided.

1. What should be filled out prior to waxing a client? _____

2. Allergies or _____ must be noted and documented.

3. Since the last time you saw them, clients may be taking new medications such as antidepressants, hormones, cortisone, medicine for blood pressure or diabetes, or such topical prescriptions as Retin-A®, Renova®, and

   _____.

4. Give clients post-wax precautions: avoid _____, exfoliation, creams with fragrance, other ingredients that may be irritating, and _____ for at least 24 to 48 hours after waxing.

5. Why should you wear gloves during a waxing service? _____

   _____

6. How can you prevent burns? _____

7. Why should you cover the scalp while performing facial waxing? _____

   _____

8. Why should you never wax over a curve on the body? _____

   _____

9. What is an alternative to hair removal if a client is contraindicated for facial waxing? _____

10. What is the angle that you should hold the spatula in for waxing? _____

EYEBROW SHAPING

Label the Image

On the first diagram below, show the point where the brow should begin and end. On the second diagram, draw the eyebrow and illustrate where the arch should be.

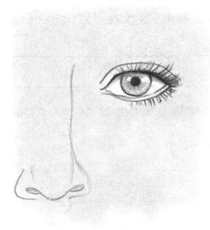

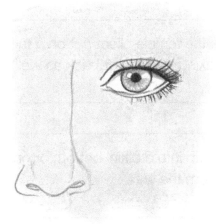

BODY WAXING PROCEDURES

Fill in the missing directions for body waxing below.

1. Use the same equipment as for the eyebrow waxing procedure, with the addition of larger strips and a larger metal or single-use wooden spatula. A metal spatula holds the heat longer, but it must not touch the client's skin as you apply the wax and must not be used if prohibited by your regulatory agency. You may find single-use spatulas more convenient. Prepare the correct strip sizes.

2. _____

   _____

3. Drape the treatment bed with single-use paper, or use a bed sheet with a towel or paper over the top.

4. _____

   _____

5. Instruct the client on how to prepare, and be mindful of her or his modesty and comfort.

6. _____

   _____

7. If waxing the underarms, have the female client put on a facial gown or wrap. Offer a wrap or towel when waxing the legs or back as well.

8. _____

   _____

9. Tuck in a paper towel or wax strip into a bikini bottom or on the edge of the pants to protect any clothing from the wax.

10. _____

   _____

   _____

WAXING TIMES AND PRICES

Short Answer

What is the estimated length and price for each of the following procedures?

1. Eyebrow _____

2. Lip _____

3. Half leg _____

4. Full leg: _____

5. Underarm: _____

6. Bikini: _____

WAXING SERVICES

Short Answer

In your surrounding towns, what is the average rate salons are charging for these services? Use at least three comparable rates for this exercise.

1. Eyebrow _____

2. Lip _____

3. Leg _____

4. Underarm _____

5. Bikini _____

HAIR REMOVAL

Word Search

Using the following word bank, write the correct word next to the definition and then find it within the word search.

anagen	hypertrichosis
catagen	lanugo
depilation	photoepilation
hair bulb	telogen
hirsutism	threading

1. The hair on a fetus; soft and downy hair. _____

2. Hair reduction methods using lasers and intense pulsed light (IPL). _____

3. Also known as banding; method of hair removal; cotton thread is twisted and rolled along the surface of the skin, entwining hair in the thread and lifting it out of the follicle. _____

4. Second transition stage of hair growth; in this stage, the hair shaft grows upward and detaches itself from the bulb. _____

5. Growth of an unusual amount of hair on parts of the body normally bearing only downy hair, such as the face, arms, and legs of women or the backs of men.

_____

6. Process of removing hair at skin level. _____
7. Swelling at the base of the follicle that provides the hair with nourishment; it is a thick, club-shaped structure that forms the lower part of the hair root.

   _____

8. Final hair-growth stage, the resting stage. _____
9. Excessive hair growth where hair does not normally grow. _____
10. First stage of hair growth during which new hair is produced. _____

```
N S G H Q R F H J N H A L K S N N L X N
X C S K C K Z X V J X N X H L E N T M O
M A N T L L A N U G O T D P G T C S H I
K N S T A N X H N H T H X A T G A J C T
X N O I T A L I P E D P N K P S U K H A
H U F N W F S V H E J A R S I C E G L L
X N H K H R N P N U Y E U S F N Q K N I
T A S X A V H M E Y M X O W N Q J E C P
U E L H I C S F E D F H M A T K G P X E
S R N K R T Z V R N C J H K P X H C N O
T X D T B M U L V I G E E H L D N S P T
M E S R U D T K R H V C T E E N F H V O
S K U M L S N T K D A U T Y Z D N D H H
I E K Q B T R Q P T T L A T J U E F U P
T K T X H E S H A S P S F R D T G U H A
U U L R P D S G R N D H U P N L O Z X E
S K Z Y K K E V F H G L E H X D L V S L
R T H T V N F X E Q Z X M H S M E H X C
I S N U S T H R E A D I N G K D T N Y Z
H S M U R E S V M J N G L X O T V D S H
```

19 Advanced Topics and Treatments

Date: _____

Rating: _____

WHY STUDY ADVANCED TOPICS AND TREATMENTS?

Short Essay

Why should estheticians study and have a thorough understanding of advanced topics and treatments? Provide answers below.

_____

_____

_____

_____

_____

_____

_____

_____

_____

_____

_____

_____

_____

_____

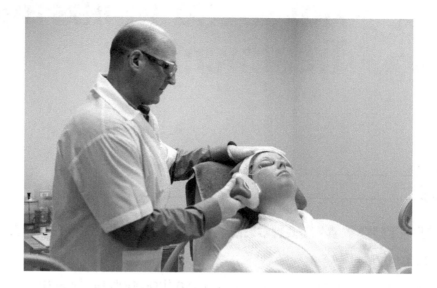

© Milady, a part of Cengage Learning. Photography by Dino Petrocelli.

CHEMICAL EXFOLIATION

Short Answer

Answer the following questions in the spaces provided.

1. What are the terms that refer to removing excess accumulation of dead skin cells?

   _____

2. What is a type of mechanical exfoliation treatment? _____

3. What can be used for a chemical exfoliation treatment? _____

4. What were the ingredients that were in the deep peel physicians used in 1882?

   _____

5. What depth of peel is a Jessner's peel? _____

6. What is a popular type of AHA that is used for peeling? _____

7. What is a popular BHA that is used to help with acne? _____

8. What type of ingredient do companies put inside their alpha hydroxy acid products to raise the pH to make the product more alkaline? _____

9. What are the benefits of a chemical peel?

   _____

   _____

   _____

   _____

   _____

10. List the 13 contraindications for a chemical exfoliation procedure.

- _____
- _____
- _____
- _____
- _____
- _____
- _____
- _____
- _____
- _____
- _____
- _____
- _____

MICRODERMABRASION

Short Answer

Answer the following questions about microdermabrasion.

1. Microdermabrasion employs the use of two procedures—crystal abrasion and _____ .

2. The benefits of microdermabrasion are: _____
   _____
   _____
   _____ .

3. What does the vacuum used in microdermabrasion stimulate?
   _____

4. What can improper use of the microdermabrasion cause?
   _____

LASER TECHNOLOGY AND LIGHT THERAPY

Short Answer

Answer the following questions about laser technology and light therapy.

1. What are lasers used for in the medical esthetics setting?

   _____

2. What do lasers emit? _____

3. What are some of the different types of lasers? _____

4. What is light therapy? _____

   _____

5. What does IPL stand for? _____

6. What does LED stand for? _____

7. What type of skin does a blue LED help? _____

8. What is photorejuvenation? _____

   _____

9. What benefit does a red LED give? _____

10. What should the esthetician and the client be wearing during a light therapy/laser treatment? _____

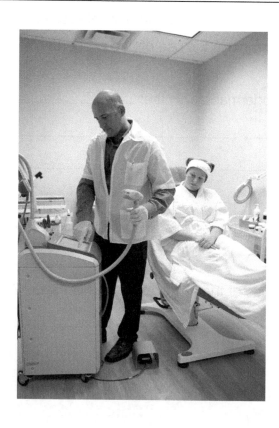

MICROCURRENT, ULTRASOUND AND ULTRASONIC TECHNOLOGY

Short Answer

Answer the following questions in the spaces provided.

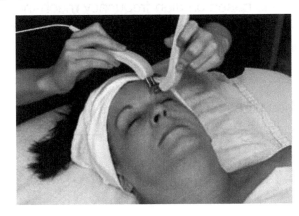

1. What is another name for microcurrent? _____

2. In the esthetics realm, what is microcurrent used for? _____

_____

3. Approximately how many sessions are needed to start with? _____

_____

4. What are the contraindications for microcurrent?

_____

_____

_____

5. Explain the technique that is used when applying microcurrent.

_____

_____

_____

_____

6. Can humans hear ultrasounds? _____

7. What are the benefits of ultrasound? _____

_____

8. How is cellulite affected by the ultrasonic technology? _____

_____

_____

9. Ultrasonic equipment is based on high-frequency mechanical oscillations produced by a metal spatula-like tool. What is the benefit of providing a procedure using ultrasonic equipment?

_____

10. What is it called when ultrasound sends waves through the skin for product penetration? _____

SPA BODY TREATMENTS

Crossword Puzzle

Put the appropriate answer to each definition in the crossword puzzle.

Across	**Clues**
1. _____	uses water in one of its three forms
2. _____	based on a system of zones
3. _____	concept based on the three doshas
4. _____	color that is sprayed on the body
5. _____	product is applied and then the body is wrapped

Down	**Clues**
6. _____	cellulite treatment
7. _____	stimulates lymph fluid to flow through the lymphatic vessels
8. _____	manual exfoliation over the entire body
9. _____	treatment of physical ailments using therapeutic water baths
10. _____	uses hot or cold stones
11. _____	re-mineralize and detoxify the body
12. _____	energy healing

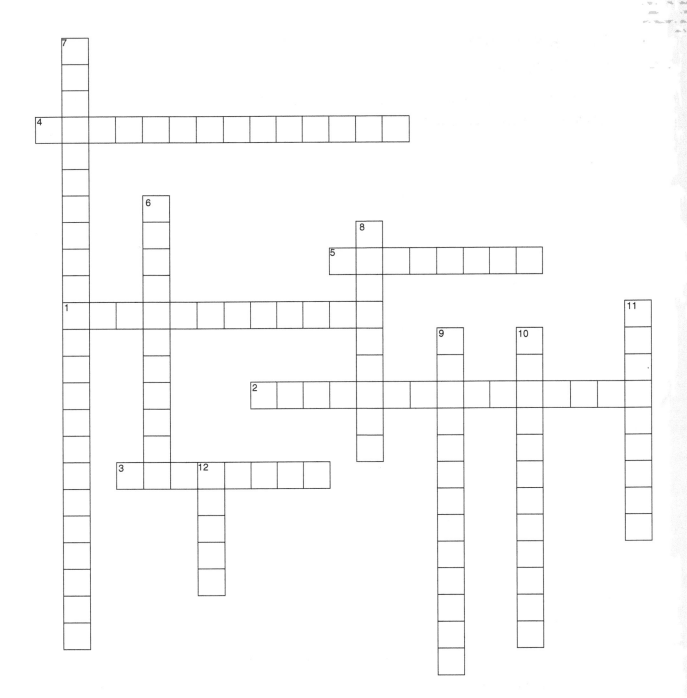

REFLEXOLOGY

Label the Image

On the foot outline below, write down the correct corresponding body parts that you would locate on a reflexology map.

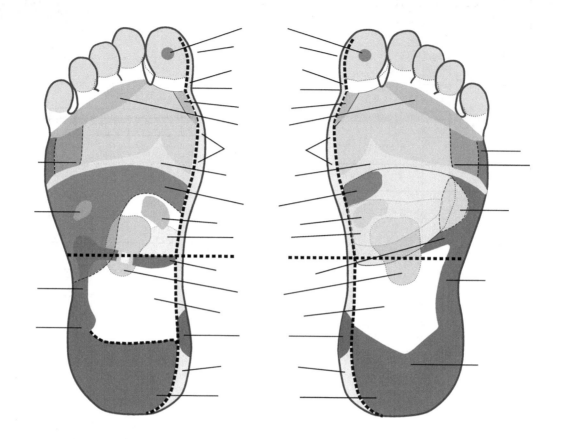

MEDICAL AESTHETICS

Short Answer

Answer the following questions in the spaces provided.

1. Explain what medical aesthetics entails. _____

_____

_____

2. What are the most popular medical spa services? _____

_____

_____

3. What are some of the treatments estheticians can do pre-operative?

_____

4. What are some of the benefits of post-operative care? _____

_____

5. What documentation should be in the patient's file? _____

_____

_____

_____

6. What is a rhytidectomy? _____

_____

7. What is a rhinoplasty? _____

_____

8. What is a blepharoplasty? _____

_____

9. Define dermabrasion. _____

_____

10. Define liposuction. _____

_____

20 The World of Makeup

Date: _____

Rating: _____

WHY STUDY THE WORLD OF MAKEUP?

Short Essay

Provide your answer as to why estheticians should study and have a thorough understanding of facial makeup.

_____

_____

_____

_____

_____

_____

_____

_____

_____

_____

_____

_____

_____

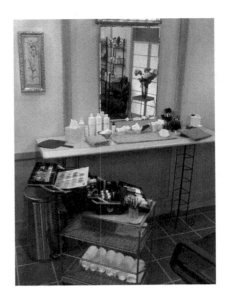

COLOR THEORY

In the following space, draw a color wheel and then identify the primary, secondary, tertiary, and complementary colors.

COLOR THEORY

Define the Term

Define the following terms in the spaces provided.

1. Define hue: _____

_____

_____

2. Define shade: _____

_____

_____

3. Define tint: _____

_____

_____

4. Define tone: _____

_____

_____

5. Define saturation: _____

_____

_____

6. Define value: _____

_____

_____

7. What are the undertones of a warm color? _____

_____

_____

8. What are the undertones of a cool color? _____

_____

_____

MAKEUP PRODUCTS AND FORMULATIONS

Short Answer

Explain what function the following products perform.

1. Foundation: _____

_____

_____

2. Mineral makeup: _____

_____

_____

3. Concealer: _____

_____

_____

4. Face powder: _____

_____

_____

5. Blush: _____

_____

_____

6. Eye shadow: _____

_____

_____

7. Eyeliner: _____

_____

_____

8. Eyebrow makeup (pencils or shadows): _____

_____

_____

9. Mascara: _____

_____

_____

10. Lip colors: _____

_____

_____

MAKEUP BRUSHES

Fill in the Blank

Fill in the missing information within the chart.

Type of Brush	Description and Use Most brushes can be interchanged and used for more than one purpose.
Powder brush	
	Smaller, more tapered version of the powder brush used for applying powder blush; can be angled.
Kabuki brushes	
	Available in a variety of sizes and ranging from soft to firm. The softer and larger the brush, the more blended the shadow will be. A firm brush is better for depositing dense color than for blending it. Small brushes are best for dark colors.
	Fine, tapered, firm bristles; used to apply liner to the eyes.
Angle brow brush	
Lash and brow brush	
	Similar to the concealer brush, but smaller and with a more tapered, rounded edge; also used to apply concealer.

PRODUCTS, TOOLS, AND ACCESSORIES

Word Search

Below is a list of the supplies needed for a makeup application. Review the list and identify them within the word search.

sponges	lash comb	spatulas
brushes	hair clips/headband	cotton swabs
lash curler	cape/neck strip	mixing cups
disposable mascara wands	tissue	

```
M A N T L L A N E C K S T R I P C S H I L A H
K N S T S N X H N H T H X B M O C H S A L C C
X N O I D A L I P E D P N K P S U K H A H K H
H U F N N F S E U S S I T S I C E G L M L F L
X N H K A R N P N U Y E U S F N Q K I I N D N
T A S X W V H S P I L C R I A H J X C P C S C
U E L H A C S F E D F H M A T K I P X E X U X
S R N K R T Z V R B C J H K P N H C N O N W N
T X D T A M U L V R G E E H G D N S P T P A P
C A P E C D T K R U V C T C E N F H V O V D N
S K U M S S N T K S A U U Y Z D N D F H S H G
I E S Q A T R Q P H T P A T N U E F U S B S U
T K P X M E S H A E S S F A D T G U B A H E H
U U A R E D S G R S D H B P N L O A X E X G X
Q K T Y L K E V F H G D E H X D W V S L S N N
R T U T B N F X Z Q A X M H S S E H X C X O A
I S L U A T H R E E D I N G N D T N Y Z A P Y
H J A I S E S V H J N G L O O T V D S H S S S
P S S K O T H R E A D G T G K D T N Y Z Y A U
L O N L P X H S E A D T N H K A T N Y Z A F S
I S Q W S T H R H A O G N G K G T N Y Z Y C O
O P H U I H H V D C D L A S H C U R L E R A Y
Z D N K D B H G Q A D G N C K D T N Y Z Y V M
```

INFECTION CONTROL

Fill in the Blank

Fill in the missing words within the basic infection control list for a makeup station.

1. Do not _____ product containers to hands or previously used applicators. Distribute onto clean palettes, brushes, or sponges.

2. _____ powders with clean brushes or spatulas onto a tissue or clean tray.

3. Scrape off powders and other products before and after use if _____.

4. Do not apply lipstick or gloss directly to the lips from the container or tube. Use a _____ to remove the product, and then apply with a clean brush.

5. If the product is accidentally contaminated, follow your supervisor's directions either to throw away the product or give it to your client. _____ put it back with your clean products to reuse.

CLIENT CONSULTATIONS

Short Essay

Write at least five questions that should be on a makeup application client questionnaire.

_____

_____

_____

_____

_____

_____

_____

_____

_____

_____

_____

_____

_____

SELECTING MAKEUP COLORS

Short Answer

Answer the questions below on selecting the correct makeup colors for your client.

1. What are the three main factors when choosing colors for a client?

   _____

   _____

   _____

2. What is the temperature of the color pink?

   _____

   _____

   _____

3. What is the temperature of the color purple?

   _____

   _____

   _____

4. If someone's skin color is light, what colors will create a more dramatic look?

   _____

   _____

   _____

5. If someone's skin color is dark, what colors will create a more dramatic look?

   _____

   _____

   _____

6. What would be a good complementary color eye shadow for blue eyes?

   _____

   _____

   _____

MAKEUP APPLICATION TECHNIQUES

Crossword Puzzle

Use the clues below to complete the crossword puzzle.

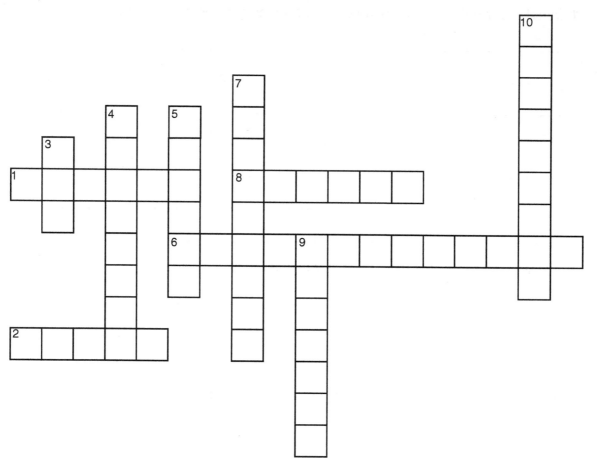

1. Lip liners are used to _____ the lips.

2. Two different color foundations can be _____ together to custom-blend a color.

3. One of the purposes of using loose powder is to _____ the foundation.

4. Foundation should always be matched as closely as possible to actual _____.

5. A contour eye shadow color is usually applied in the _____ of the eyelid.

6. When applying mascara you should use a _____.

7. Place the concealer _____ over blemishes to avoid discoloration.

8. A light shade brings out the features and dark shades causes them to _____.

9. Highlighters are _____ than the skin and contour shades are darker than the skin.

10. The technique of patting the sponge to apply foundation is also called _____.

FACE SHAPES AND PROPORTIONS

Label the Image

Fill in the characteristics of each face shape.

Face Shape	Characteristics
Oval	
Round	
Square	
Rectangle (oblong)	

© Milady, a part of Cengage Learning.

Triangle (pear-shaped)	
Heart	
Diamond	

CORRECTIVE MAKEUP

Short Answer

1. Describe how you would use the knowledge of contouring and highlighting to make a round face shape appear oval.

_____

_____

_____

2. How would you make a wide jaw appear smaller?

_____

_____

_____

3. How would you make a receded chin appear larger?

_____

_____

_____

4. How would you make a wide nose appear skinnier?

_____

_____

_____

5. How would you alter close-set eyes to have them appear a little wider apart?

_____

_____

_____

6. How would you conceal dark under eye circles?

_____

_____

_____

7. How would you create the appearance of larger eyes with someone who has small eyes?

_____

_____

_____

8. How would you create the illusion of a perfect eyebrow if a client had a shorter length eyebrow? _____

_____

_____

9. How would you correct a thin, lower lip?

_____

_____

_____

10. How would you perform a corrective makeup service on someone with a small mouth and lips?

_____

_____

_____

SPECIAL OCCASION MAKEUP

Short Answer

Answer the following questions in the spaces provided.

1. List at least four events for which a client would need specialized makeup.

   _____

   _____

   _____

   _____

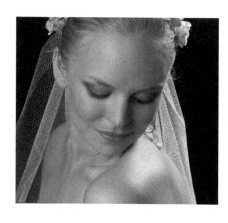

2. In what instance would someone need camouflage makeup?

   _____

   _____

3. What are the two types of artificial eyelashes that can be applied to a client?

   _____

   _____

4. What is the purpose of lash and brow tinting?

   _____

   _____

5. How long should eyelash extensions last?

   _____

   _____

6. Permanent cosmetics is also called

   _____

   _____.

MAKEUP APPLICATION

Label the Image

Using the blank diagram below, use makeup powders, colored pencils, or crayons to create a bridal makeup look.

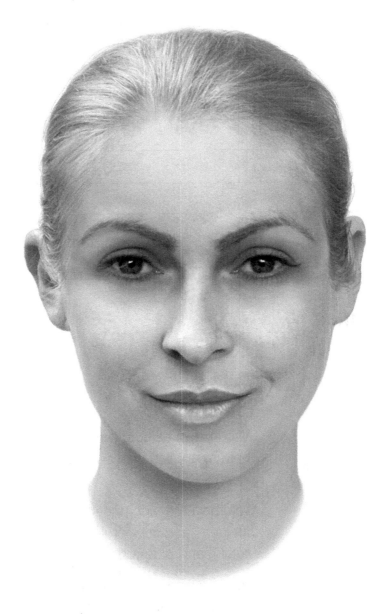

RETAILING

Short Answer

As a makeup artist, you can really raise your income by selling products. Next to the following products, write a script as to how you would sell each one.

1. Blue eyeshadow: _____

_____

2. Blush: _____

_____

3. Black eyeliner: _____

_____

4. Loose powder: _____

_____

_____

COMMON TERMS

Word Scramble

Unscramble each word by using the definition as a clue.

1. tteam   Non-shiny, dull _____

2. bdna shaels   Also known as strip lashes; eyelash hairs on a strip that are applied with adhesive to the natural lash liners _____

3. oolc locrso   Colors with a blue undertone that suggest coolness and are dominated by blues, greens, violets, and blue-reds _____

4. yrttiaer rosloc   Colors formed by mixing equal amounts of secondary color and its neighboring primary color. _____

5. uonnfaodti   Also known as base makeup; a tinted cosmetic used to cover or even out skin tone and coloring of the skin. _____

6. nepasegarit   Heavy makeup used for theatrical purposes. _____

7. ryirmap sorlco

Yellow, red, and blue; fundamental colors that cannot be obtained from a mixture.

_____

8. yee atgbnbi

Procedure in which individual synthetic eyelashes are attached directly to a client's own lashes at the base. _____

9. rcosneday csorlo

Colors obtained by mixing equal parts of two primary colors. _____

10. yotamplecmren lcorcs

Primary and secondary colors opposite one another on the color wheel.

_____

Date: _____

Rating: _____

WHY STUDY CAREER PLANNING?

Short Essay

Why should you study career planning? What are some of the things that you should consider when thinking about your own career? Provide your answer below.

_____

_____

_____

_____

_____

_____

_____

_____

_____

_____

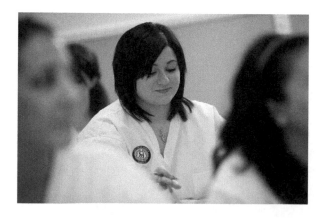

PREPARING FOR LICENSURE

Short Answer

In the space provided, answer the following questions.

1. How many hours does your state require to complete the esthetics program?

_____

2. List some tips that will help you gain control of taking your exam.

a) _____

b) _____

c) _____

d) _____

e) _____

f) _____

_____

g) _____

_____

h) _____

_____

i) _____

j) _____

_____

k) _____

l) _____

_____

m) _____

_____

n) _____

_____

o) _____

_____

3. What is deductive reasoning? _____

_____

4. List the strategies that are associated with deductive reasoning.

- _____

- _____

- _____

- _____

- _____

- _____

- _____

5. What is the purpose for a practical exam? _____

_____

6. What are two questions that you should ask yourself when preparing for employment? _____

_____

7. List the different environments where you could be employed.

- _____

- _____

- _____

- _____

- _____

- _____

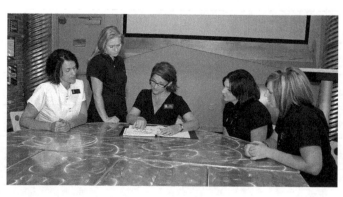

© Milady, a part of Cengage Learning.
Photography by Dino Petrocelli Photography.

RESUME WRITING

Short Essay

Write your own resume/achievements on the space below. Please refer to page 633 of your textbook for an example of a resume.

_____

_____

_____

_____

_____

_____

_____

_____

_____

_____

_____

_____

_____

_____

_____

_____

_____

_____

_____

_____

_____

_____

_____

NETWORKING

Short Answer

List the various ways you can start networking.

- _____

  _____

- _____

  _____

- _____

  _____

- _____

  _____

- _____

  _____

- _____

  _____

- _____

  _____

- _____

  _____

- _____

  _____

- _____

  _____

- _____

  _____

ON THE JOB

Matching

Using lines, match the words to the best-fitting description.

personal consideration	**1.** Maintain a clean, neat work environment and a polished personal appearance. These are important considerations in building client confidence.
prompt service	**2.** Use good manners when interacting with clients. Practicing proper etiquette is an important part of conducting yourself professionally.
professional appearance	**3.** Remember that no one wants to wait. Punctuality shows clients that you value and respect their time.
positive attitude	**4.** Give each client your undivided attention. Respectful listening demonstrates a genuine interest in the client's concerns.
courteous behavior	**5.** False claims damage the client's trust. Be sure to tell the truth when it comes to the products and services you provide.
competence	**6.** Clients need to know they can rely on your expertise. Make sure you are knowledgeable about the treatments you are practicing and the products you use. When in doubt, seek support from supervisors, manufacturers, or other educational sources.
honesty	**7.** A pleasant and helpful attitude makes clients feel welcome and cared for. If you cannot provide a particular service or certain information, make an effort to find out how the client can obtain it.

POLICIES AND PROCEDURES

Short Answer

Every salon has policies and procedures to follow. The following is a basic list of items you should be aware of when you begin your employment at a salon. Fill in the missing policies.

1. correct protocol for calling in sick or late

2. _____

3. length of vacation time and number of days that can be accrued over time

4. _____

5. _____

6. detailed job description highlighting specific duties and responsibilities

7. insurance plan and payment procedure

8. _____

9. _____

JOB DESCRIPTION

Mind Mapping

Using the mind map provided, write what you feel your ideal job could be. Write down the qualities and different aspects that you think would make it ideal.

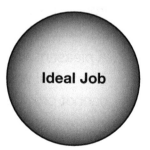

EMPLOYEE EVALUATION

Short Answer

Complete the following questions by placing your answer in the space provided.

1. What is the purpose of an employee evaluation?

   _____

   _____

2. What are three different types of compensation you can receive?

   _____

   _____

3. What do tips or gratuities express?

   _____

   _____

4. Define independent contractor.

   _____

   _____

5. Define role model.

   _____

   _____

6. Who is your role model? Why do you want to emulate that person?

   _____

   _____

EMPLOYMENT

Short Essay

In the space provided, write an essay in which you describe your idea of a great employee for a salon. If you owned your own salon, what qualities would you look for when hiring a salon professional?

_____

_____

_____

_____

CONCLUSION

Word Search

Using the word bank below, write the correct word next to the definition and then locate it within the word search.

commission	networking	salary
quota	independent contractor	deductive reasoning
resume	transferable skills	role model
job description		

1. _____ The specified list of duties and responsibilities that are required of an employee in the performance of his or her job.

2. _____ It is someone who sets his or her own fees, controls his or her own hours, has his or her own business card, and pays his or her own taxes.

3. _____ Those abilities, such as sales training or administrative skills, that were mastered at other jobs and can be applied to a new position.

4. _____ A method for gauging the amount of sales and targeting production levels.

5. _____ A method of compensation that specifies a certain amount of pay based on either a flat or hourly rate.

6. _____ A person whose behavior and success are worthy of emulation.

7. _____ A method of compensation that is percentage-based and is directly related to the employee's performance; for example, the employee earns a certain percentage of whatever services he or she performs and/or a certain percentage of the amount of product he or she sells.

8. _____ A written summary of education and work experience that highlights relevant accomplishments and achievements.

9. _____ It is the process of reaching logical conclusions by employing logical reasoning.

10. _____ It is a method of increasing contacts and building relationships to further one's career.

```
M A N T L L A N Z G O T D P G T C S H I L A H
K N S T Y R A L A S T H X B M O C H S A L R C
X N O I D A L I P E D P N K P S U K H A H O H
H U F S L L I K S E L B A R E F S N A R T T L
X N H K A R N G N U Y E U S F N Q K I I N C N
T A S X W V H N P I L C R I A H J L C P C A C
U E L H A C S I E D F H M A T K E P X E X R X
S R N K R T Z N R B C J H K P D H C N O N T N
T X D T A M U O V R G E E H O D N S P T N N P
C N P E C D T S R U V C T M E N O H V O E O N
S O U M S S N A K S A U E Y Z D T D F H T C G
I I S Q A T R E P H T L A T J U K F U S W T U
T T P A M E S R A E O S F R D T O U N A O N H
U P A T E D S E R R D H U P N L R O X E R E X
Q I T O L K E V F H G L E H X D I V S L K D N
R R U U B N F I Z Q Z X M H S S I H X C I N A
I C L Q A T H T E A D I N G S D N N Y Z N E Y
H S A I S E S C M J N G L I O T G D S H G P S
P E S K O T H U E A D G M G K D T N Y Z Y E U
L D N L P X H D E A D M N H K A T N Y Z A D S
I B Q W S T H E H A O G N G K G T N Y Z Y N O
O O H U I H H D D C D L A S H C U R L E R I Y
Z J N K D B H G Q R E S U M E D T N Y Z Y V M
```

22 The Skin Care Business

Date: _____

Rating: _____

WHY STUDY THE SKIN CARE BUSINESS?

Short Essay

What do you think are the critical points when planning and starting your own business? Provide your answer below.

_____

_____

_____

_____

_____

_____

_____

_____

_____

_____

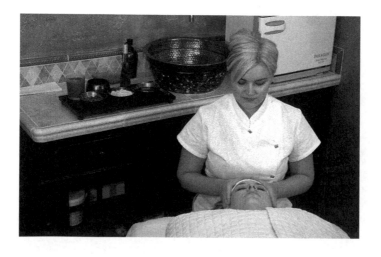

GOING INTO BUSINESS FOR YOURSELF

Fill in the Blank

In the spaces provided, answer the following questions with the appropriate word(s) or phrase.

1. To be successful, you will need to have lots of _____, a clear _____, and solid _____.

2. Booth rental allows you to experience operating a business on a much _____.

3. Renting space does not necessarily mean that you have complete control over your _____.

4. As a booth renter, you are responsible for paying all personal taxes associated with being _____.

5. Before renting a treatment room, you should find out the rate of turnover of both _____.

6. Some state boards require a special _____ for booth rentals.

7. If you are interested in attracting a high-end clientele, you should seek out a _____ area.

8. High-traffic areas provide access to a larger number of _____.

9. The _____ provides the practitioner with a strategy for understanding key elements in developing a business.

10. Before signing a lease, you should conduct a complete and thorough _____ of what other businesses are offering and the prices they are charging.

11. Hiring a professional business consultant may ultimately be the most _____ way to start up your business.

12. Your business plan should include the following:

    a) _____

    b) _____

    c) _____

    d) _____

    e) _____

    f) _____

    g) _____

13. Learning to think in terms of _____, _____, and profits can help you to gain a more global perspective of business functions as you develop your plan.

14. _____ are constant costs.

15. _____ refer to expenses that can fluctuate.

16. _____ is the money coming in.

17. _____ is the amount of money available after all expenses are subtracted from all revenues.

18. Your business must be in compliance with all _____ regulations.

19. The federal government oversees laws regarding _____ _____ taxes.

20. Although insurance may provide the business owner with a certain peace of mind, it may not protect you from _____ conduct.

21. A salon can be owned and operated by a(n) _____ _____.

22. _____ is one of the best ways that a business owner can protect his or her assets.

23. Corporations are managed by a _____.

24. Should you decide to purchase an established salon, always seek the professional advice of a(n) _____ and _____.

25. When renting or leasing space, be prepared to _____ of your agreement with your landlord.

26. To operate a successful salon, you will need a variety of _____ and _____ skills.

27. The smart businessperson recognizes that she or he _____ be all things.

28. Working from your business plan, determine how much _____ you will need to operate your business for at least two years.

29. Before you can determine the price for _____ and _____, you need to understand their value.

30. Proper service pricing begins with exact knowledge of what it costs to provide each _____.

31. To stay in business, you must learn to work _____ with your staff.

32. To attract quality and experienced help, you must be willing to offer _____ salaries and benefits.

33. The well-run salon offers _____ policies and posts these in an area that is _____.

BUSINESS TERMS

Fill in the Blank

Match the following terms with their descriptions below.

day-to-day	apprenticeship	visibility
treatments	strategic	malpractice
health	functions	accessibility
parameters		

1. Booth rentals allow the esthetician to operate a business within certain _____.

2. A booth renter is responsible for conducting all necessary business _____.

3. Some states require estheticians to complete a(n) _____ before becoming a booth renter.

4. In a booth rental situation, being the sole person responsible for all _____ operations is a big responsibility.

5. As a booth renter, you will be required to procure _____ and _____ insurance.

6. Determining the types of _____ you want to offer will help you to define your business.

7. Once you are clear about your overall business concept, you are ready to develop a _____ plan.

8. Once you have defined your target market, you can address factors such as _____ and _____.

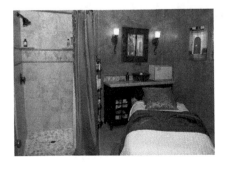

BUSINESS PLAN

True/False

Circle whether the statement is true or false, and then provide an explanation in the space below.

T   F   **1.** One of the most crucial elements in attracting business is parking.

_____

_____

_____

T   F   **2.** It is usually in your best interest to locate your salon in a high-density, high-competition area.

_____

_____

_____

T   F   **3.** It is a wise idea to develop a unique menu of services.

_____

_____

_____

T   F   **4.** One of the best ways to find your target market is to study the area's demographics.

_____

_____

_____

T   F   **5.** A business plan will help you afford the things you will need for your business.

_____

_____

_____

FINANCE

Word Search

Fill in the blanks with the correct terms. Find each term in the word search provided.

revenue	variable	capital	accountant	corporation
profit	sole proprietor	fixed	remain	initial

1. _____ is the money available after meeting all financial obligations.

2. _____ costs refer to expenses such as utilities, supplies, and advertising.

3. _____ is the income generated from selling services and products.

4 _____ costs refer to expenses such as rent and loan payments.

5. A _____ is accountable for all expenses and receives all profits.

6. One advantage to having a partnership is increased _____.

7. In a _____, taxation is limited to the salary that you draw.

8. Most buyers are concerned about the _____ return on their investment.

9. Before buying an existing salon, seek the advice of a(n) _____ and business lawyer.

10. When purchasing an existing salon, it is important to ascertain that the existing employees will _____ with the salon.

```
N S G H Q R F H J N H A L K S M N L X N
X C S K C K Z A V J X N X D L N N T M O
M A N E L B A I R A V T D E G I C S R I
K N S T A N X H N H T H X X T A A J O T
X N O I T A L P P A D P N I P M U K T A
H U F N W F R V H C J A R F I E E G E L
X N H K H O N P N C Y E U S F R Q K I I
T A S X F V H M E O M X O W N Q J E R P
U E L I I C S F E U F H M A T K C P P E
S R T K R T Z U R N C J H K P O H C O O
T X D T B M N L V T G E E H R D N S R T
M E S R U E T K R A V C T P E N F H P O
S K U M V S N T K N A U O Y Z D N D E H
I E K E B T R C P T T R A T J U L F L P
T K R X H E A H A S A S F R D T A U O A
U U L R P P S G R T D H U E N L I Z S E
S K Z Y I K E V I H G L E M X D T V S L
R T H T V N F O E Q Z X M A S M I H X C
I S A U S T N R E A D I N G K D N N Y Z
H L M U R E S V M J N G L X O T I D S H
```

LEGAL AGREEMENTS

Fill in the Blank

Using the word bank, fill in the word that best fits in the space provided.

goods	disclosure	negotiate
exemption	legal	lease
inventory	security checklist	services
unencumbered		

1. In general, a purchase agreement to buy an established salon should include:

    a) a formal written and _____ purchase and sale agreement.

    b) a complete and signed statement of _____, including all products, equipment, and fixtures.

    c) free and _____ use of the salon's name.

    d) complete _____ of all information.

2. When renting or leasing space, be prepared to _____ the terms of your agreement with your landlord.

3. When writing up a lease, allow a(n) _____ for fixtures or appliances that are attached to the salon so they can be removed without violating the lease.

4. Include the option that you can _____ your salon to another person.

5. It can be helpful to create a _____ for closing or opening the salon.

6. In general, the type of salon and clientele it serves determine the cost of _____ and _____.

THE IMPORTANCE OF KEEPING GOOD RECORDS

Fill in the Blank

Fill in the blank with the correct word(s) or phrase.

1. Keeping accurate track of daily, weekly, and monthly records will help you to determine _____.

2. Income is generally recorded as _____ from sales and services.

3. Do not forget to document any miscellaneous or cash expenses for _____ reporting purposes.

4. Small cash outlays may be kept in a _____ notebook.

5. Understanding the amount and types of services that are performed can serve as a _____ and _____ system for using products and controlling expenses.

6. Inventory can be broken down into two categories: _____ and _____.

7. Inventory and purchase records will help to prevent _____ and avoid _____.

8. Client records are instrumental in _____ the overall performance of the salon or _____.

9. Understanding what _____ and _____ clients need or want will ultimately increase sales and improve client _____.

10. In today's impersonal world, the simplest _____ can make a significant difference in how the client _____ your efforts.

Chapter 22 The Skin Care Business   **249**

FINANCIAL STRATEGY

Matching

Match the following terms with their descriptions.

net worth

manual

financial

correctly

objectives

tracking
conducting

retail supplies

trends
marketing

1. You will need to keep good records to manage your accounts efficiently and _____ .

2. A bookkeeper is trained in _____ record keeping.

3. Keeping track of daily, weekly, and monthly records is useful in assessing the _____ of your business.

4. Whether you choose a computerized program or _____ method, you will need to keep track of all sales on a daily basis.

5. _____ inventory and supplies is an important part of _____ business.

6. Accurate records can help you to determine which _____ are sold most often.

7. Analyzing accurate client records provides useful information for tracking customer _____ and performing _____ tasks.

8. Maintaining accurate client records allows you to meet your business _____ , including customer service and performance analysis

PLANNING THE PHYSICAL LAYOUT

In the space below, draw a layout of your idea of a perfect salon. Be sure to include the reception area, front desk, and retail area.

TELEPHONE SKILLS

Short Essay

1. Design a telephone introduction for all of your employees to use when answering the phone.

_____

_____

_____

_____

2. Design a telephone script for while you are having a special on a service that is offered in the salon.

_____

_____

_____

_____

_____

_____

_____

_____

_____

_____

_____

_____

_____

_____

_____

MANAGING PERSONNEL

Short Answer

Write down some of the guidelines of managing employees. The first one is written in for you.

- Honesty is always the best policy.

- _____

- _____

- _____

- _____

- _____

- _____

- _____

TRAINING PROGRAM

Short Essay

Some salons offer training programs for new estheticians. What would you want to be taught in a new salon? If you owned your own salon, what would be some of the practices that you would teach?

_____

_____

_____

_____

_____

_____

_____

_____

_____

_____

CONCLUSION

True/False

Write a T for true or F for false depending on the accuracy of the statement. If the statement is false, explain why in the space provided.

_____ 1. A booth rental is an arrangement in which the esthetician is required to pay the owner a set rental fee, along with payment of utilities as agreed upon, to operate in a specific space within the owner's establishment.

_____

_____ 2. Operating costs that are constant (for example, rent and loan payments) are known as variable costs.

_____

_____ 3. Income generated from selling services and products is called revenue.

_____

_____ 4. A form of business ownership in which two or more people share ownership (though this does not necessarily mean an equal arrangement) is known as a partnership.

_____

_____ 5. Planning and developing of relationships to achieve a certain desired behavior is called a procedural guide.

_____

_____ 6. Items available for sale to clients are known as inventory.

_____

_____ 7. A business plan is a strategy for understanding key elements in developing business; it also serves as a guide to making informed business decisions.

_____

_____ 8. The particular identifying characteristics of an area or population, such as the specific size, age, sex, or ethnicity of its residents; average income; and buying habits, are called public relations.

_____

_____ 9. Another name for employees is personnel.

_____

_____

_____ 10. A form of business ownership in which an individual is responsible for determining all policies and making all of the necessary decisions associated with running a business is called a corporation.

_____

_____

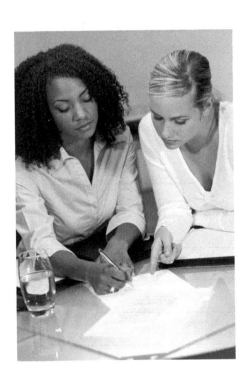

23 Selling Products and Services

CHAPTER

Date: _____

Rating: _____

WHY STUDY SELLING PRODUCTS AND SERVICES?

Short Essay

Explain below as to what you think are some of the important points to remember when selling your products and services.

_____

_____

_____

_____

_____

_____

_____

_____

_____

_____

_____

_____

_____

_____

_____

_____

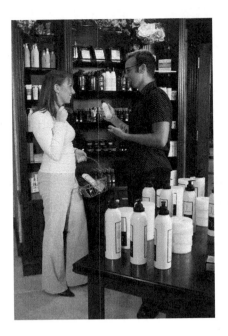

SELLING IN THE SKIN CARE SALON

Short Answer

Answer the following questions with the correct answer in the space provided.

1. In many cases, the esthetician's aversion to selling stems from negative associations that portray sales agents as pushy or aggressive people who are interested only in making money. To move beyond this negative connotation, estheticians must learn to recognize what? _____

    _____

    _____

2. In your own words, explain consultative selling. _____

    _____

    _____

    _____

3. What is the definition of retailing? _____

    _____

    _____

    _____

4. A _____ knowledge of products and services makes it easier to educate clients and increase retail sales.

5. List five points to keep in mind when selling.

_____

_____

_____

_____

_____

6. Explain the definition of upselling. _____

_____

_____

_____

_____

_____

7. What would you upsell with a facial? _____

_____

_____

_____

_____

8. Explain how you would merchandise a cleanser, toner, and moisturizer.

_____

_____

_____

_____

CONSULTATIVE SELLING

Mind Mapping

Surround the main topic of consultative selling with the 10 basic principles.

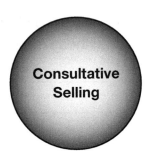

Consultative Selling

PROMOTIONS

Short Answer

There are many examples of promotions. Create a list of some of these examples. Some of the answers have been provided for you.

1. Use seasonal themes and holidays to promote packages at special prices.

2. _____

_____

3. _____

_____

4. _____

_____

5. Demonstrate customer appreciation by giving clients a discount or complimentary service during their birthday month.

6. _____

_____

7. _____

_____

8. _____

_____

9. Offer discounts or add value to services on slower days.

10. _____

_____

11. _____

_____

PROMOTIONS

Draw two different pieces of promotional material that you can have for your own business.

MARKETING

In the space below, create an advertisement for your salon.

CLIENT VALUE

Short Answer

It is always important to have the client fill out the intake form and for you to not only store their pertinent information but also add some of your own notes. List 8 pieces of information that you should store. The first one is filled out for you.

- Name

- _____

- _____

- _____

- _____

- _____

- _____

Your awareness of these details will make them feel important. Include the following information on client records:

- _____

- _____

- _____

- _____

CLIENT RETENTION

Fill in the Blank

Fill in the missing words in the following guidelines that help maintain the professional expertise of an esthetician and benefits clients derive from quality skin care treatments.

1. Continually provide quality service. Once you have won a customer over, it is easy to become complacent. To avoid this common pitfall, estheticians must work hard to maintain their skills and provide excellent service all the time.

2. Understand what the client wants, and _____. Never forget that each client has a unique agenda. Always set aside time to update information and address client concerns. This lets clients know you are genuinely interested in understanding and fulfilling their individual skin care needs.

3. Give each client your personal, undivided attention. Again, everyone wants to feel special. Get in the habit of treating clients as if they are special guests. _____ Offer refreshments and practice proper salon etiquette.

4. Develop good listening skills. There is no substitute for the genuine respect that comes from actively listening to another person. _____ _____ will encourage clients to share their concerns openly. This will enable the esthetician to provide a more effective treatment plan.

5. Give clients incentives to _____ Most salons specifically train the front desk staff to rebook clients. Without the esthetician's support, however, clients may view this as just another sales tactic. Encouraging clients to book their next appointment is a good way to let them know you are dedicated to improving the condition of their skin. Keeping them informed of any special offers or programs that can save them money is also a good way to show that you have their best interests at heart.

SUCCESS

Short Answer

Answer the following questions in the space provided.

1. What is one of the most important roles that an esthetician has that happens after the treatment? _____

_____

_____

2. How do you keep track of your success? _____

_____

_____

3. Now that you have a better understanding of the esthetics field, what would be

your ideal place of business? _____

_____

_____

CONCLUSION

Word Scramble

Determine the answer to the following question by unscrambling each word, using the definition as a clue.

sandgvertii

1. Promotional efforts that are paid for and are directly intended to increase business.
_____

iecnlt edcorr epgekin

2. A method of taking personal notes that helps the esthetician to remember important data and better serve client needs.
_____

liectn olcnostuntai

3. An opportunity at the end of a treatment session to review product recommendations, prepare a home-care program for the client to follow, and provide any additional literature on other treatment options that the client may be interested in. _____

nsvcultiaote lelnlisg

4. A method of advising or consulting to clients and recommending the best treatments and products for their use. _____

ermchasndgiin

5. This is how retail products are arranged and displayed in your salon. _____

nopmiorto

6. The process of getting the consumer's attention with the goal of increasing business.
_____

piucylibt

7. Free media attention. _____

qeaiuneorsnti

8. This is the form that provides the esthetician with a complete client profile. _____

rntelaiig

9. The act of recommending and selling products to clients for at-home use.
_____

guspnleli esrisvce

10. The practice of recommending or selling additional services to clients that may be performed by you or other practitioners in the salon. _____